THE FEEL-GOOD HOME

Feng Shui and Taoism for Healthy Living

MARY JANE KASLINER

THE FEEL–GOOD HOME

Feng Shui and Taoism for Healthy Living

Mary Jane Kasliner

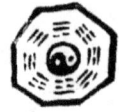

Text © by Mary Jane Kasliner
Interior Illustrations © by Ann Curch Gagliano
Registered in the Library of Congress
Interior and cover formatting by Rend Graphics www.rendgraphics.com

Paperback ISBN: 978-0-578-65057-9
Revised 2025

All rights reserved. No part of this book may be reproduced or utilized in any form or by any means, electronic or mechanical, including photocopying, recording or by any information storage and retrieval system, without prior permission in writing from the publisher.

This book is solely for educational purposes. Even though this book may provide a connection between health problems and the environment, anyone in need of medical assistance should consult a healthcare practitioner.

The author nor the publisher can accept responsibility for any damage or injuries caused directly or indirectly by the information contained in this book.

"Learn as though you would never be able to master it; Hold it as though you would be in fear of losing it."

Confucius

"We must always change, renew, rejuvenate ourselves; otherwise we harden."

Johann Wolfgang von Goethe

Table of Contents

Acknowledgements — vii
Foreword by Yasha Jampolsky — viii
Introduction — x
List of Figures — xii

Chapter 1: The Origin of Feng Shui — 1
- Chinese Philosophy & Principles of Feng Shui
- Observation of the Heavens
- Land Formations

Chapter 2: The Ch'i of Life — 13
- What is Ch'i
- Cosmic Ch'i, Human Ch'i & Earth Ch'i
- Directionology
- Auspicious & Inauspicious Ch'i

Chapter 3: Yin Yang & The Five Elemental Energies — 25
- The Concept of Yin & Yang
- The Tai Chi Symbol & Seasonal Changes
- Yin Yang, Five Elements & The Human Body
- 5 Elemental Foods
- Birth Elements & Your Environment

Chapter 4: The Connection Between Earth Energies, Man-Made Energies & Disease — 53
- History of Ley Lines
- Dowsing
- Electro-Stress & Disease
- Electromagnetic Frequencies in the Home
- Protective Measures

Chapter 5: The Human Living Space — 73
- Selection of House Sites & Land Assessment
- Attacking Shapes & Structures
- Human Body Perspective in the Home
- Architectural Shapes & Structures

Chapter 6:	The Symbolic Bagua	113
	• Building the Trigrams	
	• Superimposing the Map of Life	
	• Health & Family	
	• Wealth & Resources	
	• Self Confidence & Reputation	
	• Relationships	
	• Creativity	
	• Helpful People	
	• Career	
	• Wisdom	
Chapter 7:	Designing The Essential Rooms for Health	129
	• Dwelling Compatibility	
	• The Impact of Clutter	
	• Guidelines for Healthy Design	
	• Remedies for Problematic Spaces	
Chapter 8:	Consecrating Your Space	157
	• What is Space Clearing	
	• Building Energetics	
	• Space Clearing Procedures	
	• Creating a Sacred Space with Geometric Forms	
Chapter 9:	Alignment of Mind, Body & Soul	173
	• The Auric & Chakra Systems	
	• Balancing the Chakras with Crystals & Stones	
	• Essential Oils to Balance the Aura & Chakras	
	• Meditation	

Epilogue: 191
Appendix: 193
    12 Zodiac Signs of Western Astrology
    12 Animals of Eastern Astrology
    About the Author
    About the Illustrator

Resources & Bibliography 207
Additional Notes 213

Acknowledgements

First, I must recognize the ancient sages and their dedication to the development of Feng Shui. Because of their efforts, future generations can utilize the principles to obtain the utmost contentment and prosperity.

I am grateful for my teachers whose commitment has allowed me to learn this fascinating and complex subject. Without them I would never have seen the changes unfold in my life and the lives of my clients.

I express my gratitude to my colleagues, many of whom are authors on this subject matter, who didn't hesitate to share their expertise and perspective on the principles of Feng Shui.

I would also like to express my appreciation to my students who are always optimistic and eager to learn the history and science of Feng Shui. Many of them have gone on to be wonderful consultants themselves.

Many thanks to Ann Curch Gagliano for her amazing illustrations throughout this book. Her talent for interpreting concepts and transforming them into works of art is extraordinary.

Thank you to my daughter Christina for her patience and support while I worked on this project. I deeply appreciated her assistance during the final stages of putting this book together.

My heartfelt praise to my wonderful husband Ron. His kindness, support, and encouragement were a constant source of inspiration and motivation in undertaking the awesome project of writing this book.

In conclusion, I would like to thank those interested in studying Feng Shui. I encouraged them to share their newfound knowledge. I hope that we all can experience life filled with health, harmony, and prosperity.

Namaste,

Mary Jane Kasliner

Foreword

Written by Yasha Jampolsky

I began as Mary Jane's teacher and sometimes Mentor. We ultimately became good friends and fellow travelers on road to scholarly awareness. Upon hearing of this book I expected great things and have not been disappointed. This book is full of essential and practical wisdom and also explains some advanced principles of Feng Shui. It is also filled with exquisite artwork making it a delight to the eyes and very suitable as a gift that almost anyone would enjoy.

I first met Mary Jane several years ago when she enrolled in a class at the New York School of Feng Shui. I was a Director at the time. I was quite surprised to see her there since I knew she had already completed a Certification Program at another school. I later learned that this was not unusual for her because her insatiable thirst for knowledge and joyful pursuit of learning was a lot of what she was about. It is this that has led her to become most knowledgeable in so many areas that reflect and influence the field of modern Feng Shui.

Later as a student in my Four Pillars training program, Mary Jane stood out again. Her thoughtful questioning of the subject matter and her ever inquisitive interest in the deepest and most subtle aspects of the material presented, was an ongoing inspiration to the class and to me, as instructor.

As the title explains, this book focuses on the methodology of living our healthiest lives. Ancient Taoist thought predicates that health be held above all else. To achieve our best and healthiest state requires an understanding of the elements that bring the required balance and lead to a harmonious existence. There are obvious and subtle influences that come to play in the achievements of these ends and these are well delineated in this book, especially as they pertain to our living environment.

This book offers a history of Feng Shui as well as a plethora of tools and methods. Some are easy to learn and some require a little work to master. Whether you desire to achieve mastery or would like to know the basics, you will find the content of this book fascinating and effective.

Foreward written by Yasha Jampolsky

It covers such a broad range of subject matters that you are bound to find personal alignment somewhere within its pages.

In my over thirty years of involvement with healing energy work and Asian studies I have encountered magnificent teachings and exceptional teachers. I believe that there is a new generation of inspired individuals who have studied the ancient wisdoms and have combined them with the realities of modern life and the essential connections to spirit. In this category, I believe, Mary Jane is at the front of the pack.

I continue to be impressed with Mary Jane's limitless capacity for knowledge, impeccable integrity, and consummate passion whether as a Feng Shui Consultant, Educator or Author.

Yasha Jampolsky - is an Educator, Author and Consultant in Feng Shui and Four Pillars Chinese Astrology. He has appeared on radio and national television and is a regular contributor to Feng Shui and lay publications. He offers training and certification in the New York Metropolitan area and nationally.

Introduction

Writing a book is no simple feat. It requires levels of motivation, commitment, and patience to endure a process that can be painstakingly arduous at times. In order to succeed in such a project, I believe you must have passion for the subject matter and the desire to share your passion with others.

For me, the study of Feng Shui is that passion. After twenty years of working in medicine and dentistry, I finally have found my soul's mission. In 2000, I discovered this ancient Taoist philosophy and immediately found its subject matter intriguing – the laws of nature, the cosmos, and topography of planet earth. My insatiable desire to further educate myself about its principles and practice has been relentless throughout the years. I still find myself constantly yearning for more knowledge today, and I am sure for many years to come.

At the core of all Feng Shui lies the subtle beauty of nature; all of its essence exudes a level of harmony and balance unparalleled. It is man's premise to experience the Heavens and Mother Earth for all they have to offer. It is not until we are finally able to do so, that we can then obtain life's most divine gifts.

It is my intention for readers to not only understand the components of Feng Shui, but also how the ancient sage and astronomer discovered concepts of time, direction, seasons, and energies of the earth from them. With knowledge of these concepts, the ancients constructed cities, palaces and dwellings in a way to obtain maximum levels of health, vitality and prosperity. Total well-being is attainable by merely respecting nature and living in unison with it. Unfortunately, in this day in age, the majority of us have removed ourselves from nature. We live in structures that drain us physically, mentally, and spiritually and as a result lose our focus and soul's purpose. Feng Shui offers the necessary means to reconnect ourselves with nature, fellow man, and heavenly energy.

Today, Feng Shui practitioners around the world incorporate its age-old principles to balance the surrounding environment in ways that instill health and harmony. Throughout the pages of this book, you will discover how the core concepts of Feng Shui are applicable to modern day architecture and how the use of sacred geometry nurtures the sensory body. By incorporating higher vibrations of nature into our homes, we align our personal energy, awaken our inner selves, and unlock our soul's missions. Balancing our environment with Feng Shui ultimately allows us to regulate our physical, mental and spiritual attributes to create complete harmony.

My avocation lies in teaching others how to create a healthier and more successful living environment for themselves by reconnecting to the divine forces of the Universe. I hope you will join me in this celebration of years of education, hard work, and discovery by opening yourself up to the principles that have withstood the grueling tests of time. By embracing its ideas, Feng Shui can show you that we all have the unlimited power to attain our life's ambitions, but we must first choose to let them in.

Mary Jane Kasliner

List of Figures

Figure 1:	Hetu Map	2
Figure 2:	Earlier Days Ba-gua	2
Figure 3:	Tortoise Markings	3
Figure 4:	Later Days Ba-gua	3
Figure 5:	Shipan	7
Figure 6:	Cosmograph	7
Figure 7:	Four Celestial Animals Compass Points	9
Figure 8:	Four Celestial Animals House Position	9
Figure 9:	Yin and Yang Movement	12
Figure 10:	Cycle of Sun Directional Points	27
Figure 11:	Sun Chart	27
Figure 12:	Yin and Yang Symbol	27
Figure 13:	Five Ch'i Powers	36
Figure 14:	Five Element Transformation	36
Figure 15:	Eastern And Western Zodiac Signs	40
Figure 16:	Chinese Birth Element Chart	42
Figure 17:	Trapazoid Lot	77
Figure 18:	Inverted Trapazoid Lot	77
Figure 19:	Corrugated Lot	78
Figure 20:	Triangular Lot	78
Figure 21:	Meat Cleaver Left Quadrant	79
Figure 22:	Meat Cleaver Right Quadrant	79
Figure 23:	Three Door Entry Ba-gua	92
Figure 24:	Compass School PaKua	92

List of Figures

Figure 25:	Magic Square	113
Figure 26:	Ba-gua	117
Figure 27:	L-Shape Building	118
Figure 28:	T-Shape Building	118
Figure 29:	U-Shape Building	118
Figure 30:	S-Shape Building	118
Figure 31:	East—West group	129
Figure 32:	Auspicious and Inauspicious Directions	130
Figure 33:	House Groups and Trigrams	131
Figure 34:	House Aura	158
Figure 35:	Stones For The Chakra and Aura	184
Figure 36:	Chakra Sounds and Mantras	187
Figure 37:	Chakra Oils	188

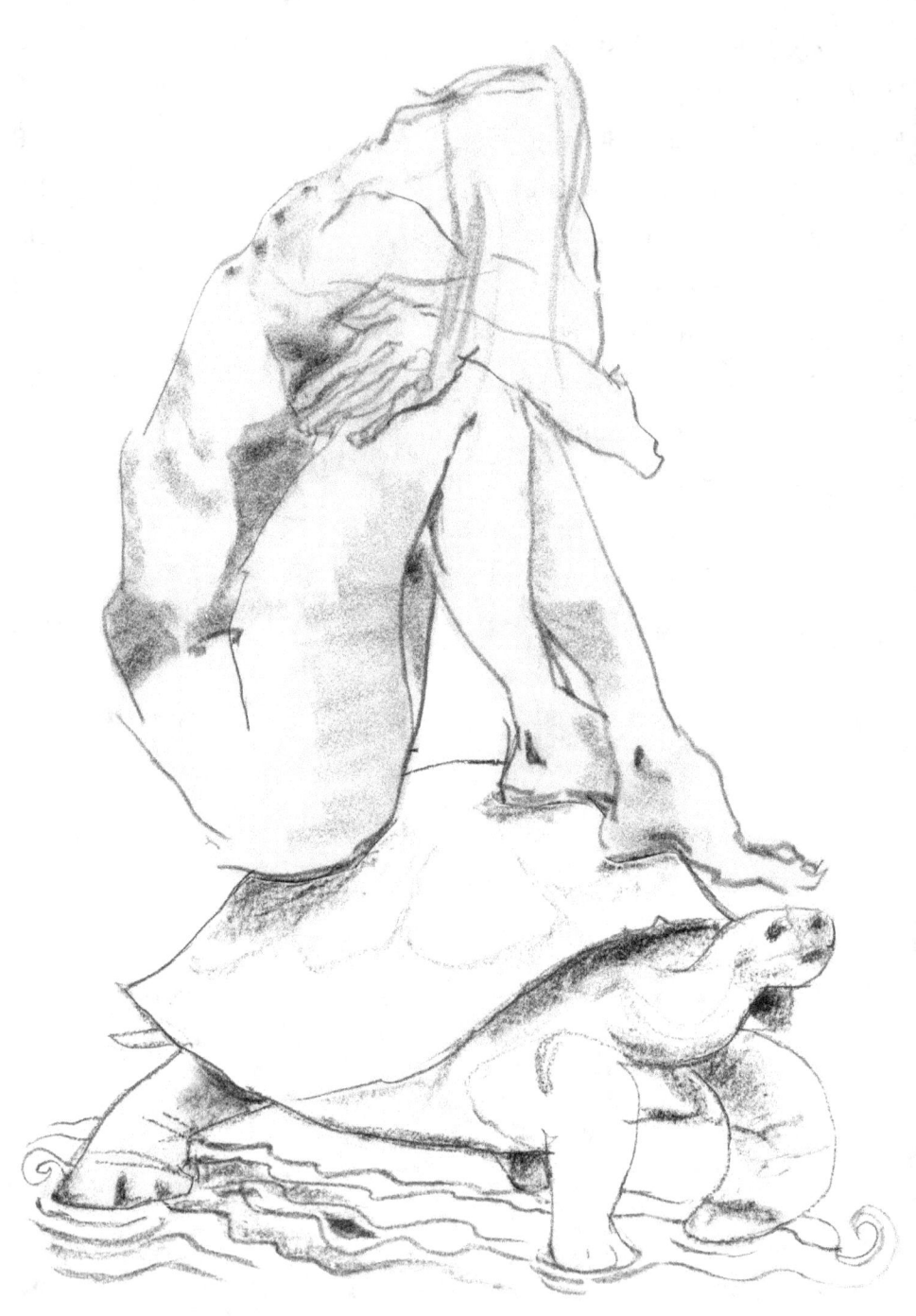

1
The Origin of Feng Shui

"What is not fully understood is not possessed."

Johann Wolfgang von Goethe

Feng Shui is an ancient practice based on Chinese philosophy. It literally means wind and water, a basis for two fundamental forms of life energy. Why Wind and Water? Because these two forms of energy act as vehicles to transport and cultivate the cosmic breath of life known as ch'i. Specifically, the wind carries this life force ch'i and the water collects, cultivates, and stores it. The wind is a result of a combination of our planet's rotational movement through space and weather patterns created by high and low pressure systems interacting. Water is an essential element of matter that is responsible for all things including solids, liquids, and gases. It is the sustaining element for life that makes up seventy percent of the surface area of this planet and seventy percent of the human body.

A large part of feng shui theory is about studying life force energy or ch'i. How this energy moves within our environment and what type of impact it has on us individually is the quintessential point behind this discipline. In order to fully understand the dynamics of feng shui, the connection between man and nature, and why the Chinese utilize these concepts, begins with understanding the Chinese culture and philosophy.

In the Chinese language there are two characters that define the word culture: Wen, meaning civilization and Hua, meaning transformation. By examining these words we can see this is a culture about transformation or change. It is a culture based on three directives: Material Goods, Human Relationships, and Spirit or Heart. The interpretations of these three cultural directives are as follows:

1. <u>Material Goods:</u> This is considered to be the essential items for sustaining life.
2. <u>Human Relationships:</u> This refers to the interaction and socialization of people.
3. <u>Spirit or Heart:</u> This is our need to express ourselves to others.

The Feel-Good Home :: Feng Shui and Taoism for Healthy Living

Although all three aspects are necessary, the emphasis is placed on the third level. It is the key aspect to bringing the harmonious whole or Tai Chi into one's life.

History

The Chinese culture spans some 5,000 years. Much of the advance knowledge in disciplines such as astrology, astronomy, mathematics, geometry, architecture and feng shui found its way to China as a result of the mass migration from Sumeria from the legendary cataclysmic flood. This mass migration led to infiltrations to all parts of the world, particularly South America, Africa, India and China. There were five distinct wandering tribes that colonized specifically in China. One of the main tribes was Fu Xi, named after Emperor Fu Xi. He was considered semi-divine and credited with teaching others how to hunt for food, farming techniques, and developing the basis for mathematics and geometry. He was further noted for establishing the eight trigrams and positioning them in an arrangement known as the Pre-Heaven or Earlier Days ba-gua that represented the Universe in perfect polarity. This was based on the intricate markings observed on a mystical horse that arose from the River Ho. It was believed this configuration of black and white dots (see below) was a divine message. Further development of this theory was based on a configuration discovered by Yu the Great on the shell of a giant tortoise. This configuration brought forth the Later Days ba-gua, commonly used in feng shui practice today. This arrangement of the trigrams presented as an ebb and flow, or dynamic and receptive movement between the cosmos (macrocosm) and the earth (microcosm).

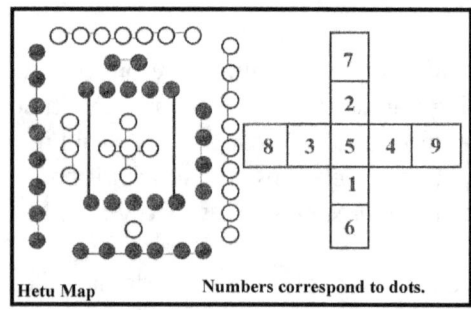

Hetu Map   Numbers correspond to dots.

Fig. 1

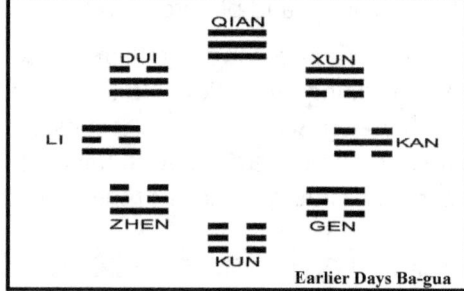

Fig. 2

Black Dot: Yin   Even #'s: Yin   Underlying Reality of the Universe
White Dots: Yang   Odd #'s: Yang

The Origin of Feng Shui

Fig. 3

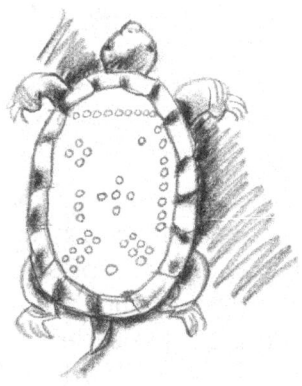

Fig. 4

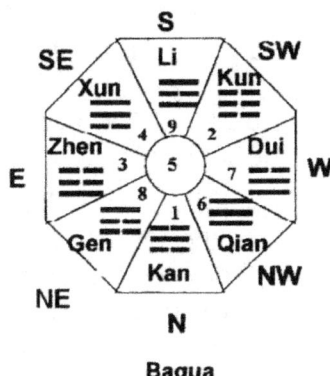

Bagua

Markings on Tortoise Progression to Bagua   Later Days Bagua-Constant Movement

By the end of the Han dynasty Confucius and Lao Tzu entered the main stream of Chinese culture. It was a time when Taoism and Buddhism had been introduced as a philosophy and religion. Confucius was considered to be a teacher of moral behavior and political ideology. Much of Confucius philosophy was based on the Golden Mean, which was derived from the I Ching. The Mean relates to the center—in a sense meaning centering oneself and not overindulging in any one thing in life. The concept of sincerity is also expressed in the Golden Mean and is said to come from the self, bringing with it enlightenment.

Lao Tzu was noted for his great book (Tao Te Ching), a basis for Taoism. Where Confucius emphasized social order and an active life, Taoism was based on the individual, nature, and tranquility. The principles were based on the laws of yin and yang and the enveloping circle of the Tai Chi, making three elements in totality. Whereby Yin is one (1), Yang is two (2), and Tai Chi is three (3). This translates into Heaven, Man, and Earth. Together they symbolically form nature. All is interconnected and thus a core balance of yin and yang exists. This can be demonstrated as:

          Heaven
          Man
          Earth

If one is to fully understand Chinese philosophy, then the I Ching should be studied. It is considered to be a classical book containing thoughts and principles of life. It is a book that assists man in opening his mind. Some of the classics noted in Chinese civilization is the Bible, The Fo Jing (or Buddhist Sutra), and The Wu Jing or Five Books. It is in the Wu Jing that the I Ching is most noted.

I (Yi) in Chinese means change. In the classical book, I Ching, there are graphics of the Sun and Moon, the ultimate yang and yin symbols of the heavens. These two luminaries represent the constant flux of energy within the Universe, as one replaces the other in a cyclical pattern. Much like man himself is in a constant state of change and growth cycles from birth to death, so too is the universe in a constant state of growth and transformation. The I Ching is simply a guide to assist man in a life of balance and harmony. When man is able to conceptualize and perceive these laws and apply them to his environment, the result is great joy and abundance in life. All Chinese philosophy is based on the concept of Tao, yin and yang, and the five elements, including Chinese medicine.

The I Ching contains sixty-four hexagrams that are built from the eight trigrams. These eight trigrams relate to the eight basic images or phenomena among us. These images are as follows: sky, earth, thunder, wind, fire, water, mountain, and marsh or lake. These images were depicted in bit language or symbols. A straight line (-) represented those things in nature that represented motion, elevations, hard and strong images. This straight line became known as yang energy. A broken line (--) represented things in nature that are motionless, depressions, soft and weak images. These broken lines came to be known as yin energy. Each of these eight images are depicted in the building of yin and yang lines known as a trigram. Each trigram tells us about how life works and how to master it. They are depicted on the ba-gua or life map.

If we begin by assessing the symbolic trigram of the eight images based on the aforementioned qualities of yin and yang, we observe the following.

```
═══
═══     Sky: Notice the three yang lines. This indicates a great
═══     power or divine being. The sky is closest to the heavenly
        points making this trigram an appropriate image.
```

The Origin of Feng Shui

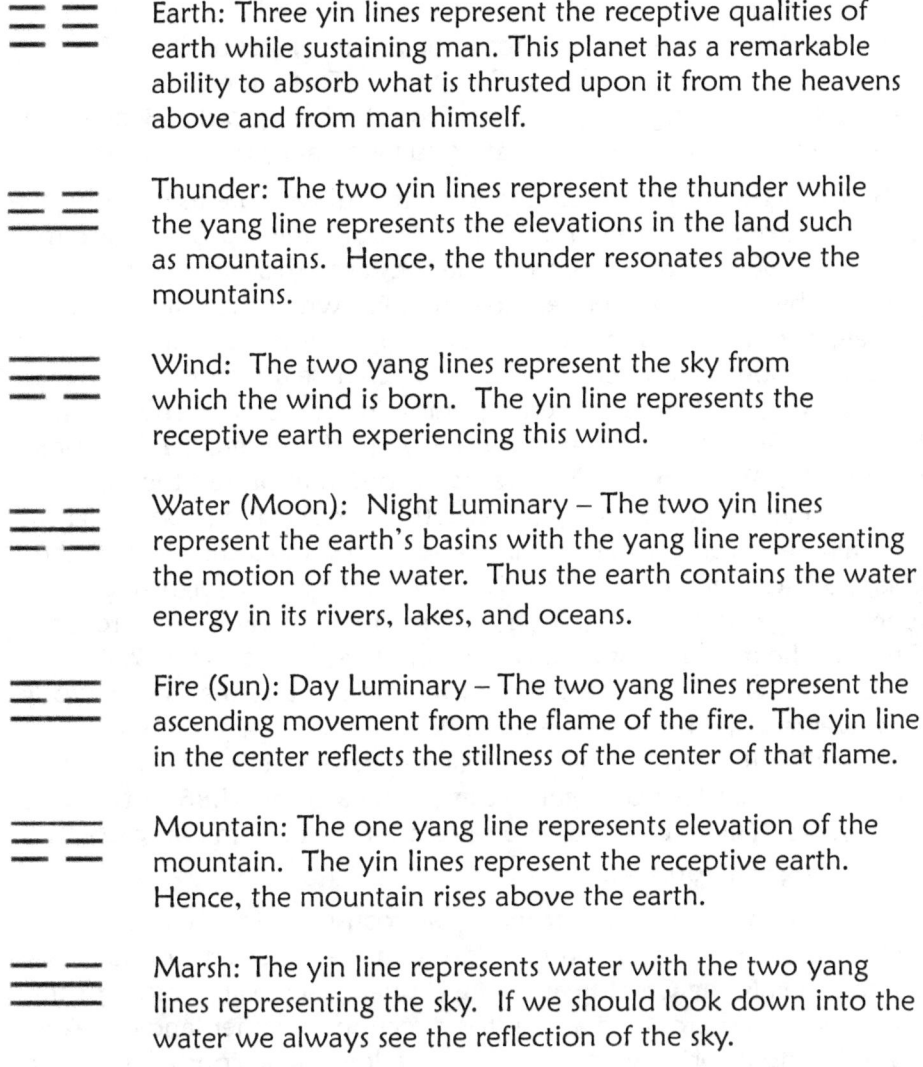

Earth: Three yin lines represent the receptive qualities of earth while sustaining man. This planet has a remarkable ability to absorb what is thrusted upon it from the heavens above and from man himself.

Thunder: The two yin lines represent the thunder while the yang line represents the elevations in the land such as mountains. Hence, the thunder resonates above the mountains.

Wind: The two yang lines represent the sky from which the wind is born. The yin line represents the receptive earth experiencing this wind.

Water (Moon): Night Luminary – The two yin lines represent the earth's basins with the yang line representing the motion of the water. Thus the earth contains the water energy in its rivers, lakes, and oceans.

Fire (Sun): Day Luminary – The two yang lines represent the ascending movement from the flame of the fire. The yin line in the center reflects the stillness of the center of that flame.

Mountain: The one yang line represents elevation of the mountain. The yin lines represent the receptive earth. Hence, the mountain rises above the earth.

Marsh: The yin line represents water with the two yang lines representing the sky. If we should look down into the water we always see the reflection of the sky.

These eight images are defined from the viewpoint of the ancient sages observing nature. The Chinese were very astute when it came to observing the interacting forces between the heavens (Astrology) and the earth (Geomancy). These observations naturally segued into theories of how man interacted with these forces.

The practice of feng shui takes into account the influences of cosmology on the earth. Therefore, the ancient sages had to have a handle on Astronomy as well as Geomancy. This is the basis for the two major schools of feng shui: Compass School relating to the Heavens or Astronomy and Form School, relating to Geomancy or land formations.

If we begin with Compass School feng shui we note its origin to the Chinese astronomer. Their method of locating stellar positions is different from their Western counterparts. The Western astronomer locates stellar positions by using a main reference point known as the ecliptic. The Chinese refer to this as the Yellow Path. This is essentially the path that the Sun, Moon, and other planets trace. Chinese astronomers use the celestial North Pole as a reference point with the celestial equator as a base line referred to as the Red Path. Due to this difference in mapping the heavens, Western astrology bases its computations on the movement of the planetary bodies along the ecliptic or zodiac (i.e.: zodiac signs) and the Chinese astrologer places prime importance of calculations on the lunar zodiac. Therefore, the sky is divided into twenty-eight segments representing one segment per day of the moon's movement through the sky. The moon takes 28 days to complete a cycle. The Western zodiac uses twelve signs to represent the months and the Chinese zodiac uses twelve animals to represent the years (i.e.: Rat, Tiger, Ox, etc.). This is called the Jupiter cycle that takes approximately twelve years to complete, as Jupiter's planetary year is equivalent to 11.86 or twelve earth years. This becomes a core calculation method in many Compass School feng shui formulas.

Chinese astrology and astronomy are considered to be one study. It takes into account many constellations that their Western counterparts do not, mainly the Great Bear or Big Dipper. The main reason for this is the big dipper provided a basis for direction on either land or sea and was referenced for seasonal changes. In addition, all constellations were considered celestial deities and the tail of Ursa Major was regarded as the "Sword of God."

By determining the directional position of Ursa Major through an instrument known first as the Shipan and then the Cosmograph, one could determine the time of day, seasons, weather patterns, when to plant crops, and many other things.

The Origin of Feng Shui

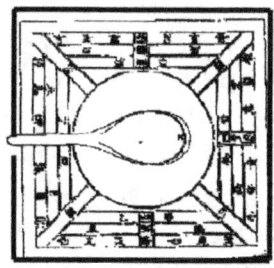

Fig. 5 **Shipan:**
Spoon handle aligns with tail of Big Dipper

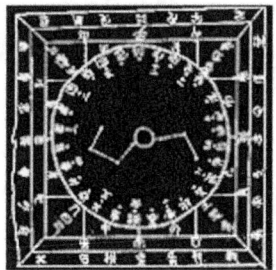

Cosmograph: Fig. 6
Big Dipper in center

The Cosmograph contained a square plate representing earth and the concept of order, and a round dial containing the configuration of Ursa Major (representing heaven). Hence, the cosmology symbol is a circle inside a square. This Cosmograph later developed into the intricate Chinese compass known as the LoPan used by feng shui practitioners throughout the world.

Since the Chinese interpreted the information received from the heavens as messages from the divine, they utilized the celestial bodies to configure their cities. By using a gnomon (vertical pillar or stick) to mark the rising and setting points of the sun, and drawing a circle on the ground to mark the midpoint of these two shadows, one could determine the axis of the earth pointing directly to the pole star. This was considered to be a point where heaven and earth meet, the four seasons merge, and where yin and yang are in harmony. The North-South axis became the alignment point for all capitols and major imperial buildings to be built, as they would directly receive the heavenly blessings. It was also believed that Beidou (Great Bear/Big Dipper) was a template used to design the entire city around.

The Chinese astronomer continued to map the heavens as this is how the celestial deities would reveal its intentions to mankind. Part of the mapping process revealed four major constellations that divided the sky into four quadrants that aligned to the four Cardinal directions.

These four major constellations are known as the Phoenix to the South, White Tiger to the West, Black Tortoise to the North, and Green Dragon to the East. Within each of these four major directional constellations are seven minor constellations, or what is referred to on the LoPan compass as the twenty-eight lunar mansions. It was said that these four celestial deities came down from the heavens and became land formations that surrounded the burial site to protect the ancestors while making their journey to the spiritual plane. These four landforms are the major components of Form School feng shui that is still practiced today.

The landform topography consists of the coiled Dragon to the East or left of a building. It represents yang or male energy and allows the entering ch'i to enfold the structure. Since the East represents the location of the rising sun, this animal is considered the most yang and is where the yang ch'i is generated and flows beneath the earth. It is important that vegetation is grown here and should grow higher in proportion to the West, or right side of the structure. The coiled Dragon can be represented in nature by tall trees, high and long mountain ranges, or buildings in cities.

The crouching White Tiger sits to the West or right side of the structure. It represents yin or female energy and allows the stagnate ch'i to roll out and away from the building. The White Tiger is considered to be the most yin of all the animals. It is noble and courageous, but also can be vicious and determined. Therefore, the West or right side of the structure should never be higher than the East or left side, as the male energy of the home will be attacked causing ill health. Lower trees, hills or buildings are all good representations of the WhiteTiger.

The hovering Phoenix bird is positioned to the front or South of the building and represents a spreading out of space allowing ch'i to enter. It is preferable that a flowing stream or fountain is positioned here to help cultivate the incoming ch'i from this direction. This area is considered the Ming Tang, or open area with a view. There should never be an obstacle such as a building, high trees, or a mountain to obstruct the view and incoming ch'i source.

The Origin of Feng Shui

The Black Tortoise sits to the North or rear of the building. The Tortoise is a sacred symbol in the Chinese culture and signifies strength, support, longevity, and tenacity. The occupants of the home or building are graced with these characteristics when the Black Tortoise is supporting the structure. Mountains, tall trees, high fences, rocks, or buildings all provide the support necessary to hold in the auspicious modulating ch'i and overall stability for the occupants.

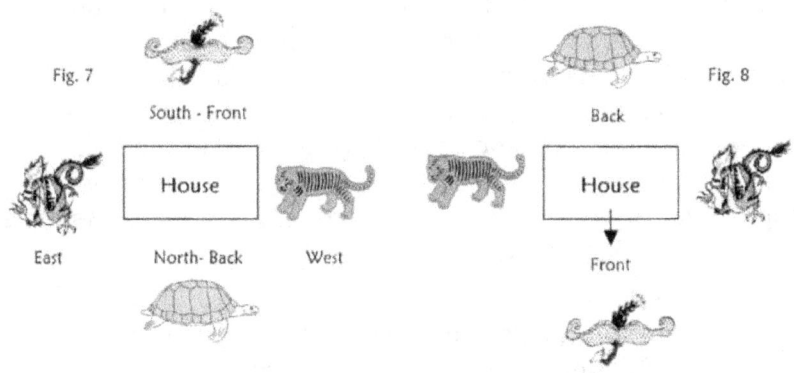

Compass Points based on sun movement   Standing inside looking out

By and large, these land formations are not aligned in compass direction with modern day feng shui. This is because homes and buildings have their own directional facing positions, whereas traditional Chinese dwellings and structures were aligned with their facing point to the South due to geography and climate. Therefore, the entrance point to the building determines the positions for the aforementioned land formations. When you stand inside the building with your back towards the building looking out, the Dragon is to the left and the Tiger is to the right. The hovering Phoenix should always be to the front with the Black Tortoise to the rear. Occupants living in dwellings that are enfolded with these landforms tend to experience high vitality, wealth, and prosperity.

Other aspects of Form School feng shui entails finding the "Earth's Ch'i" and understanding how it flows. This is referred to as following the "Dragon Veins." Just as we seek to open energy points within our body's Meridians to improve health, the feng shui master looks to locate auspicious sites for dwellings to feed the occupants with healthy ch'i.

Since water is the blood and breath of the earth's ch'i, then where water flows on the surface, ch'i flows beneath. Once the flow of water is discovered, then the point where it pools and accumulates is considered advantageous. This is pointed out in the Taoist book called the "Zhuangzi" in chapter 22: "Man's life is the assembling of qi. The assembling is deemed birth; the dispersal is deemed death." Therefore, this pooling of ch'i resonates to the assembling process.

Ch'i will follow the earth's terrain flowing within ridges and branches in the earth. The mountains are considered the acupuncture points on the earth and where the dragon resides. The hills act as a buffer for fast moving ch'i slowing it down to a proper pace. Of course there are other earth energies such as magnetic fields that flow within the earth. These fields are necessary and were recognized by the Chinese early on when the compass was invented. We can then conclude the Chinese believed ch'i had an electromagnetic quality about it.

The ability to understand the dynamics of landform and how the energy moves beneath the ground we walk upon is a science in itself. The ancient sages mastered the art of Geomancy (earth terrain) to cultivate their villages in order to sustain a life of prosperity. Today, we can incorporate these same principles to find the most auspicious location for our dwellings. By truly understanding the relationship between nature and man, we are able to connect with the heavens and earth to obtain health, harmony, and abundance. The first Taoist principle states, "There is not just us or just nature, but both." Throughout the pages of this book, we will discover how the co-dependent relationship between man and nature is responsible for our life's experience.

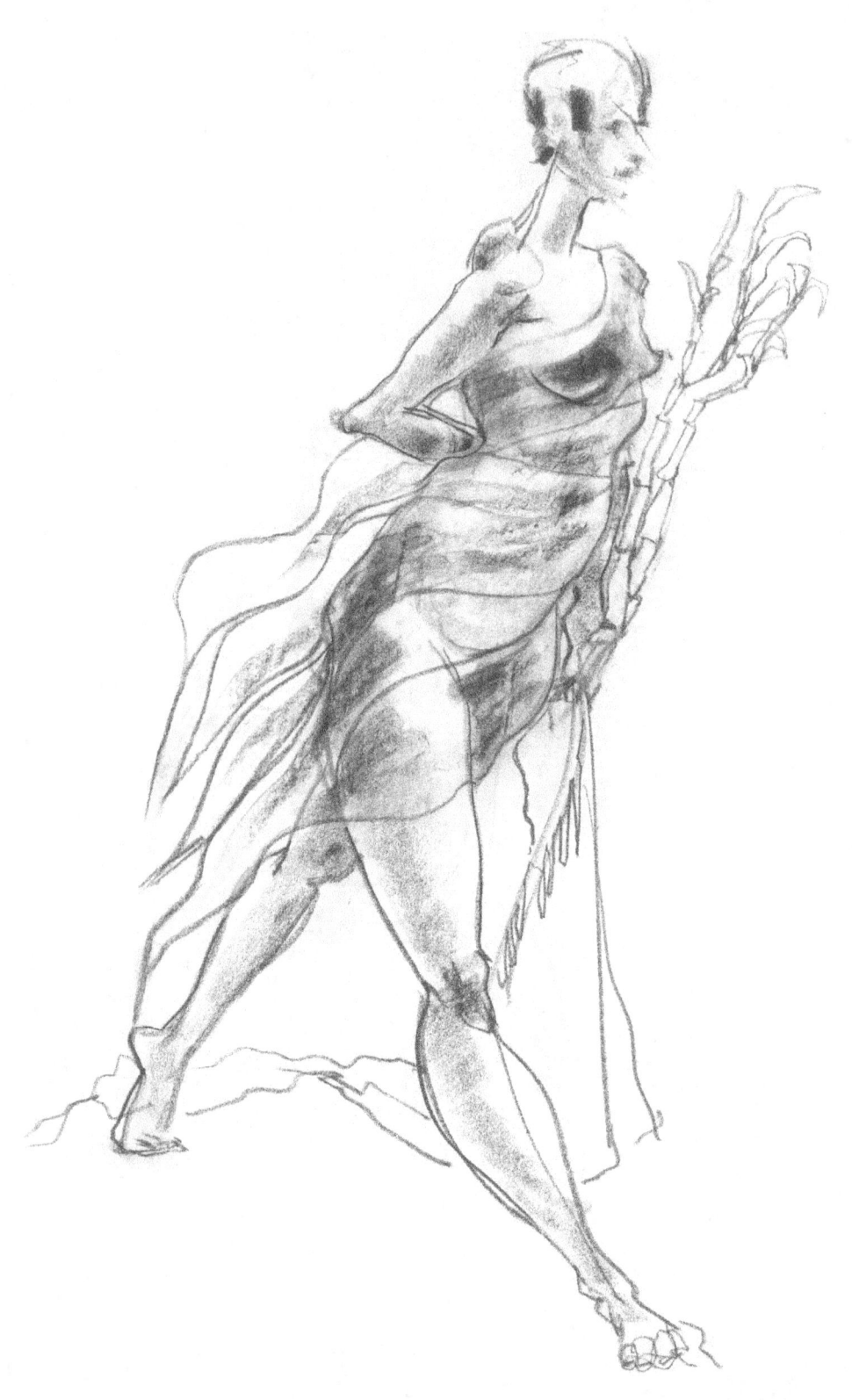

2
The Ch'i of Life

"Every Human being is the author of his own health or disease."

Buddha

Ch'i is the universal breath of life. It is the invisible energy that animates all living things flowing through the heavens, earth, and nature until it reaches our living and working spaces. It is the fundamental concept behind feng shui that links everyone and everything in the universe. The Taoist philosopher believes man is a co-worker in this universe and not the dominating master. Man has his place in the grand scheme contributing his own unique ch'i to the world.

To gain a full understanding of ch'i, one needs to go back into the annals of Chinese culture and Taoist thinking. Taoism means "The Way" and has its roots entrenched in Chinese medicine. Here, the laws of nature are observed and correlated to the unseen workings of the human body to maintain health and cure disease. The concept is based on two interdependent polarities (yin and yang) that drive the forces of the universe. Yin defines the receptive female qualities. It equates to the waters that flow on earth and the earth itself. Yang energy reflects the dynamic qualities of the male. It defines the fire that ascends to heaven and heaven itself. The constant movement and interaction of these two energies (heaven and earth) results in the creation of all things and emanates the sustaining ch'i life force. According to the laws of nature described from the Taoist perspective, yang energy always follows the yin energy. Therefore, in the schematic below we begin to see the interaction between these great forces.

Fig. 9

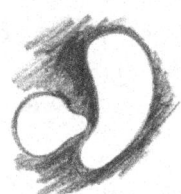

Yang-Male
Oxygen

Yin-Female
Ch'i

The concept of ch'i can be further understood through Einstein's theory of relativity ($E=MC^2$). In his theory, energy forms matter and when matter is dispersed it creates energy again. Hence, the Taoist concept that ch'i is in a constant state of flux and contained in all things is substantiated by Einstein's theory.

The Taoist philosophy also states that in order for total health to ensue there must be harmony and balance between the forces of yin and yang, the five core elements (fire, earth, metal, water, wood), and the three ch'i treasures. These treasures are made up of Heaven's ch'i, Man's ch'i and Earth's ch'i.

Heavens Ch'i

Heaven's ch'i or cosmic ch'i is the result of minute particles that drop into the earth's atmosphere from a combination of the planetary and solar rays. It governs the seasons, weather and climate, and as a result influences man directly.

To illustrate this point, let's evaluate the impact seasons have on ch'i. In the spring ch'i will take on a fresh quality, a bright energetic feel, and have a bold characteristic. The vegetation begins to purge through the earth and a sense of vitality fills the air. The ch'i is building a yang dynamic energy. As spring blossoms into summer the ch'i is at its highest yang point radiating outward, and vegetation is in full bloom. Summer gives way to autumn as yang ch'i energy begins to wane and yin ch'i slowly builds. The earth pulls inward and contracts to prepare for the long winter ahead. Vegetation is waning and works its way back into the earth. At this point the ch'i reaches its ultimate yin point and begins to build yang energy preparing for the rebirth of spring. These are the four seasons that we recognize and experience internally and externally. However, the ancient Chinese master configured a more detailed perspective of the seasons derived from their observations of nature and the cosmos. A division of twenty-four ch'i seasons marked solar, climatic, and agricultural patterns. This was essential to guide the farmer in an agricultural year. Each of the twenty-four points relates to fifteen degrees movement of the sun corresponding to fifteen or sixteen calendar days. In essence, this form of measurement gave a clear picture of ch'i growth and decay necessary for the farmer.

The climate and weather patterns we choose to live in will also directly impact our own ch'i and as a result our overall vitality and health. The Chinese believed that extreme weather patterns were unstable and therefore destabilized human ch'i. Overly cold and wet conditions caused diseases of the joints, whereas extreme heat caused conditions of the cardiovascular system. We can all associate with this premise, as many of us venture into a warmer climate during the cold winter days, or cooler weather when it is overly hot. Our bodies are very sensitive to weather patterns and always look for homeostasis to balance itself internally.

Human Ch'i

Human ch'i is the second treasure recognized by the Taoist philosopher. It is a personal and unique quality that determines your attitudes, behaviors, feelings, moods, and how you interact with others. A portion of this is the result of the position of the planetary bodies overhead at the time of birth. A Bio-psycho-science theory referred to as imprinting suggests that the constantly changing electrical energy emitted from the planets elliptical spin is imprinted at the moment of birth onto our own electro-chemical make-up. How is this possible? Humans are essentially very electrical in nature. This is because our bodies are comprised of seventy percent water and several elements including saline. Nerve impulses branch out throughout our bodies into synapses and allow neural impulses to occur. Once we are born and the umbilical cord is cut, our brain begins to function without the support of the mother's body. It is at this time the infant brain becomes a receptor to these electrical charges emitted from the planets and the earth's own magnetic field. The imprinting theory, by and large, is the basis behind the field of astrology, which makes a connection between the planetary cycles and the corresponding energies seen in earthly events and human behavior.

Human ch'i is also believed to flow throughout the body along the meridians or channels that feed the physical systems (organs) and the states of consciousness (emotions, spirit) through the chakra and auric systems. When disease is present, it is believed there is a blockage in one or more of these channels limiting the amount of ch'i energy to feed the area. This can be directly correlated to an environment that has stagnated ch'i within the land or living space. A close evaluation of the soil, various earth energies, electromagnetic fields, and the internal environment is essential for total healing of the body to occur. Otherwise, the body will continue to be subjected to sha (unhealthy) ch'i and the desired results will not be achieved.

The auric and chakra systems interface constantly with the environment expanding and contracting to adjust itself. It inhales the vibration of ch'i in color, materials, sounds, scents, objects, and shapes. Therefore, the condition of your surroundings will directly influence whether you are healthy, sickly, happy, unhappy, fortunate, or misfortunate.

To illustrate this point, let's examine the impact color has on the human body. When an environment has a great deal of browns it exudes a sense of structure. The body will respond by feeling grounded, but it also can be physically and mentally rigid. This is magnified if the furniture is a heavy dark brown wood, as there is an overwhelming feeling of authority, responsibility, and order. This is the type of ch'i then swirling about in the space and as a result infused into the human body. Colors such as yellow or orange are very uplifting and invigorating. Yellow being a stimulant to mental activities, while orange being more playful and joyful. Color is a very powerful ch'i source and an excellent healing modality for the human body. Meditations to improve physical and emotional health can be done visualizing specific colors. We will see in chapter 9 how to align the chakras using colors for overall well-being.

The types of materials you surround yourself with also has an impact on the type of ch'i you subject yourself to. For example, placing a lot of Granite stone within your environment will emit a harsh energy. It is not to say you can't place granite in your home, it simply means to balance the décor with softer elements to absorb and balance the ch'i.

The objects and symbols displayed on your walls program the ch'i either in a positive or negative way. In other words, you should choose your symbols and images carefully, as the auric system acts like a magnet drawing to it like energy. Let me explain this concept further. Your environment paints you directly and you paint it back. Therefore, if the colors, sounds, scents, symbols, and images are positive, uplifting, and in alignment with your goals in life, then this is what you will attract to yourself. On the other hand, if your environment lacks color, if it is cluttered, or contains objects and images you do not have a connection with, then this is the type of energy you will attract into your life. It sounds rather non-descript and that makes for

The Ch'i of Life

difficulties in achieving your goals.

When it comes to sounds and scents these energies have a very high vibration and as a result healing power. The human body needs to stimulate all of its senses in order to be in harmony. Keeping in alignment with the Taoist principles, observe nature for a few hours and notice the sounds and smells. This is what you need to bring into your living and working environment. Essential oils, chimes, nature sounds in the form of music, and water features are all excellent accoutrements to enhance your space and body.

The shape of objects, architecture, and clutter all impact the type of ch'i that modulates. By and large, ch'i should meander like that of a gentle stream or breeze. This is the type of ch'i the human body understands and accepts freely. When objects form right angles, whether it is from a piece of furniture or the configuration of the furniture, another building, or architectural shape of a room, the ch'i has difficulty modulating around it. As a result, a portion of the ch'i will continue onward spiraling out of control until it meets resistance and absorbed. That resistance could be you, and over a period of time this can result in aches and pains in the area that is absorbing the direct hit. This is very apparent in rooms you spend a great deal of time in since the spiraling ch'i is a repeated infraction to the specific body area. The key is to place something between it and you to absorb the out of control ch'i source. For example, by simply placing a plant, decorative throw, mirror, or something red will respectively absorb, redirect, and draw in the problematic flow of ch'i.

Just as blocked meridian channels within the body will choke vital ch'i from feeding that particular area in the body, clutter will shut down the ch'i source from meandering to that specific part of your home. When you consider the theory that every part of your house reflects a part of your body and an area of your life (see chapter 5), then the concept of stagnating ch'i caused by clutter has a greater impact. If ch'i cannot modulate and becomes stuck, you will feel the repercussions pertaining to a particular part of your life and body part. Less is more is a concept to live by. So get rid of the clutter and over abundance of furniture within your space. It not only creates chaos that will compromise your level of harmony, but brings your own energy down and keeps you stuck in the past.

Your personal ch'i is also affected by the food you ingest and the water you drink. Foods that are organically grown and not tainted with chemicals or hormones have a high ch'i source that will keep your internal ch'i and body systems functioning properly. On the other hand, foods and beverages that contain sugars, preservatives, and fillers have depleted ch'i and will deplete your own vital ch'i source. In Chinese medicine, certain foods and herbs can assist body systems and act as a healing aid. This premise is based on the five ch'i powers of expression (fire, earth, metal, water, wood) as well as yin and yang. Each element is associated with a particular color and organ system. Therefore, foods that are a certain color or that feed the particular element (birthing cycle) can be ingested to aid in the healing process. In addition, ch'i increases in the body when alkaline foods are ingested. This is because the body tends to be more alkaline than acid. Some examples of alkaline and acidic foods are listed below.

<u>Acidic Foods:</u>

- Eggs
- Liver and other organ meats
- Gravy
- Wine
- Yogurt
- Corn
- Beans
- Fish
- Fowl
- Most Grains
- Coffee

<u>Alkaline Foods:</u>

- Bananas
- Chocolate
- Figs
- Mineral water
- Orange juice
- Potatoes
- Spinach
- Watermelon
- Turnip greens
- Dandelion Greens
- Most fruits & vegetables

<u>Directionology:</u>

Directionology influences the type of ch'i that enters a home or particular room and impacts our personal ch'i directly. Historically, the Chinese refer to the directions as five cardinal points and eight directions. The five points align with the apparent movement of the sun in the sky (East, South, West, North) and the center, which is considered to be a stationary point or the ground we stand on (Earth). The eight directions reflect the eight compass points (4 cardinal & inter-cardinal) and directly corresponds to the eight trigrams and their attributes. In this section, I will discuss the eight compass directions and how aligning oneself to the supportive directional ch'i can mitigate potential challenges.

The eight directional ch'i energies are extremely powerful in how one behaves and operates. By assessing the important points within a home beginning with the front door and moving onto the kitchen, bedroom, and potential home office, we can determine what the impact of these directional points will have on the occupants. One simple way to determine what direction these rooms fall into is to take a compass and stand in the center of your home and mark off the eight directional points on a floor plan. You are then able to determine the rooms that are in the directional ch'i you are looking to absorb.

Following the sun, we begin in the East and the season of spring. The Eastern wood ch'i energy is filled with growth and potential. It represents the rising sun, activates the individual, and is the catalyst for new ideas. Things happen in this direction, as it corresponds to the thunder image in the ba-gua. Rooms that are located in this direction will feel fresh and bright motivating you to start the day and any new projects you have in mind. This ch'i is wonderful for young couples that are starting out in life, but lacks the partnering energy associated with the Southwestern ch'i.

If we continue across the sky to the Southern cardinal point, morning gives way to noon and spring blossoms into summer. This is the most dynamic ch'i energy of all the directional points, as it corresponds to the fire element. The South is imbued with the ecliptic band that houses the Sun, Moon, and planetary bodies. Needless to say, these are very powerful energies that paint this directional ch'i. Spending time in rooms with this type of ch'i will easily facilitate any projects you take on. This is the kind of ch'i that allows ideas to come to the forefront bringing with it the warmth of the sun, light, and harvest.

As the sun appears to move across the sky, summer gives way to autumn and the high point of the sun descends into the horizon. The Earth begins to pull into itself to prepare for the upcoming winter. This is the Western metal ch'i direction that is imbued with the energy of completion. It represents the end of the day, romance, relaxation, and a time to reap all that was produced.

Rooms that fall in this direction are very relaxing and great for completing projects. However, since the sun in its descent, the light source becomes de-ionized and as a result can be rather draining. The key is to inject some color back into this light source by placing a refracting crystal or stain glass ornament in the window. When the sunlight passes through the crystal or stain glass a rainbow of colors will cascade throughout the room.

Northern water ch'i is rather quiet and still like a cold winters night. It lacks the support of the direct sun, as the sun is predominantly in the southern half of the sky throughout the year. This direction can be very challenging and present with life struggles and obstacles. Since it faces the stellar, it represents long-term goals, the seeking of knowledge, and the journey to success. Slow and steady wins the race, but many times this energy feels overbearing because of a lack of patience. The positive aspect of this type of ch'i energy is its soothing and calming quality. Therefore, if you need to calm yourself down, this is a good directional energy to spend time in. The process begins again with the night turning into early morning and the winter moving into early spring. Here the earth is working overtime to prepare for the re-birth of spring.

The aforementioned are the cardinal directions representing the four seasons and ch'i fluxion. The inter-cardinal directions depict the season's gradual movement and represent a mix ch'i expression. If we begin with the Southeast, it represents mid-morning and late spring into early summer. The Southeastern wood ch'i combines the warmth and ease of the South with the activating Eastern energy. This type of ch'i activates the individual in a self-satisfying way. It is great for communicating ideas since the wind image of this direction (on the ba-gua) can carry the ideas to others.

The Southwest represents the late summer into early fall and late afternoon into early evening. It combines the warmth and ease of the Southern ch'i with the relaxing energy of the West. This direction is connected to the soil energy and as a result this ch'i is very caring and feeling in nature. Coupled with the romantic ch'i energy of the west, this becomes a great direction for the couple.

The Northwestern ch'i represents late fall into early winter and the evening hours. It is a ch'i filled with maturity, responsibility, and leadership qualities. The combination of a challenging Northern ch'i with that of the Western romantic and completing ch'i energy could present obstacles for the couple or projects at hand.

The Ch'i of Life

The Northeastern direction represents late winter into early spring and the early morning hours. There is a quick changing energy about this direction since the earth is churning beneath in preparation of spring. Therefore, it aids in decision-making and competitive situations. It also can be challenging for the individual, as there is a combination of difficult Northern ch'i with the self-actualizing Eastern ch'i.

Earth's Ch'i

The third and final ch'i treasure is Earth ch'i. It is the forces of the landscapes, mountains, rivers, plains, and valleys that accumulates and disperses ch'i. The ancient Chinese sages also referred to this type of ch'i as the arteries and veins of the dragon. Landscapes with high hills exposed to strong winds and fast moving streams were considered inauspicious because ch'i is scattered. Areas such as those collect too much yang energy and therefore considered a poor choice for building a dwelling. Landscapes with low-lying valleys and pools of water encourage ch'i and an overall quiet feel. In feng shui, water is considered an auspicious element that attracts and cultivates ch'i. This is why a water feature should be positioned to the front of a property. However, the size and movement of the water flow does make a difference. Water sources that move very quickly can over power human ch'i and therefore are considered inauspicious. Since all land in feng shui is considered mountain or water energy, in order for harmony and balance to ensue, these landforms should be present. The Mountain energy represents a still yin ch'i as it stands with its majestic appearance and stability. Water is dynamic in movement, and therefore represents yang energy. A balance of these two ch'i energies constitutes harmony and is considered auspicious for a dwelling.

To establish an environment that is supportive and nurturing, ch'i assessments should begin outdoors. A survey of the land is paramount, as strong Form School Feng Shui will provide the solid foundation for sheng ch'i to propagate and thus bless the occupants.

Begin with assessing the soil. Is it rich in nutrients to support lush vegetation? If it is, then you know it will sustain life. What is the air quality? Is it fresh and filled with negative ions or has the ch'i been transmuted from pollutants of nearby factories, highways, or an airport. How does the land present itself? Are there sinkholes, an over abundance of pine trees, or vegetation that seems to die off quickly? These are all indicators of potential underground water and electromagnetic discharges respectively. Do you notice an abundance of ants, bees, spiders, Oak or Willow trees on the property? These are all indicators of possible Geopathic Stress lines running beneath the land. What is the positioning of the property or dwelling to the roadway? Cul-de-sacs, T-junctions, Y-junctions, and blading roads will send bulleting ch'i directly to the property and the dwelling. This can cause undo stress for the occupants resulting in an array of problems from arguments, divorce, illness, etc.

Finally, assess the traditional Form School typography of the land. Is the dwelling or future dwelling enfolded with the supportive Tortoise in the rear to provide strength, tenacity, and longevity for the occupants? Is the left side or Dragon position higher than the right or Tiger side? If it isn't, then the ch'i will be rather rambunctious and thwart the male energy of the home. Is there an open view or established Ming Tang in the front to allow the ch'i to enter and feed the dwelling? If not, the ch'i is compromised by a blocking force and can present as challenges for the occupants. If you choose a property that supports, nurtures, and protects you, it becomes the fundamental basis for your overall health and success in life.

You are constantly being engulfed with different kinds of energy, whether it is from the Heavens, Earth, or others around you. How you decide to work with this energy will ultimately dictate how you experience life. If you choose to be in alignment with these energies, you will begin to tune into the universe and feel as "one." The ultimate choice is yours.

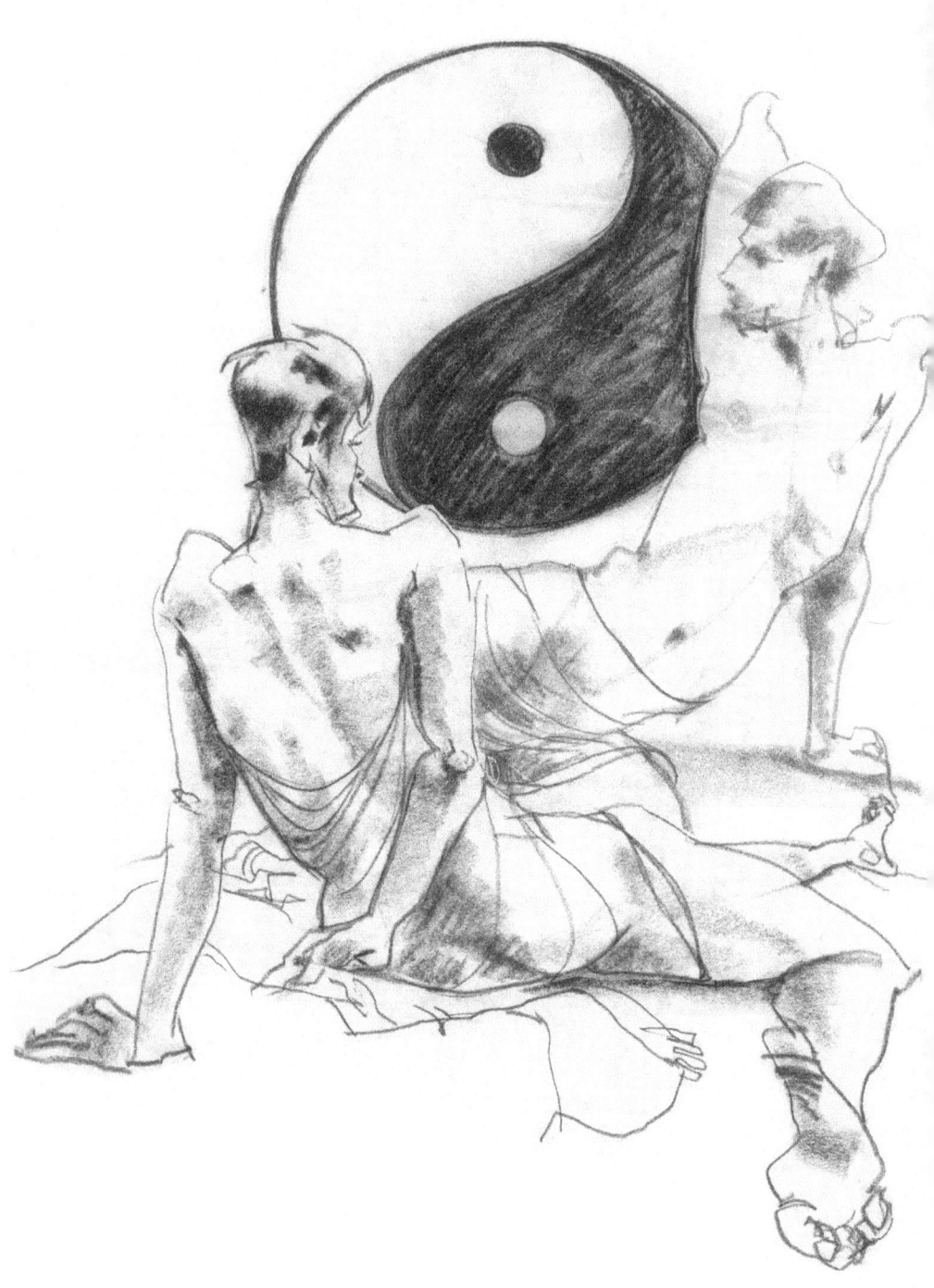

3
Yin–Yang & The Five Elemental Energies

"All things come out of the One and the One out of all things."

Heraclitus, 500 B.C.

*T*he earth was without form, and void; and darkness was on the face of the deep...Then God said, "Let there be light; And there was light...And God divided the light from darkness. God called the light day, and darkness He called night...Then God said, "Let there be firmament, and divided the waters which were under the firmament... And God called the firmament Heaven... And "Let the waters under the heavens be gathered into one place, and let the dry lands appear;" and it was so. (Genesis – Bible).

Before Heaven and Earth had taken form all was vague and amorphous. Therefore, it was called "The Great Beginning." The Great Beginning produced the universe. The universe produced material forces which had limits. That which was clear and light drifted up to become Heaven, while that which was heavy and turgid solidified to become earth. (Sources of Chinese Tradition).

Then God said, "Let there be lights in the firmament of the heavens to divide the day from the night; and let them be for signs and seasons, and for days and years; "And let them be for lights in the firmament of the heavens to give light on earth;" and it was so. Then God made two great lights; the greater light to rule the day, and the lesser light to rule the night. He made the stars also. God sent them in the firmament of the heavens to give light on the earth. Then God said, "Let the earth bring forth grass, the herb that yields seed, and the fruit tree that yields fruit according to its kind, whose seed is in itself, on the earth;" and it was so. Then God said, "Let the waters abound with an abundance of living creatures, and let birds fly above the earth across the face of the firmament of the heavens." (Genesis-Bible).

The combined essences of heaven and earth became yin and yang, the concentrated essences of yin and yang became the four seasons, and the scattered essences of the four seasons became the myriad creatures of the world. After a long time, the hot forces of the accumulated yang produced fire and the essence of the fire force became the Sun; The cold force of the accumulated yin became water and the essences of the water became the Moon. The essence of the excess force of the sun and the moon became the stars and planets. Heaven received the sun, moon, and stars while earth received water and soil. (Source of Chinese Tradition).

"The Tao begets the one, The one begets the two, The two beget the three and the three beget ten thousand things. All things are backed by the shade, faced by the light and harmonized by the immaterial breath." (Lao Tzu: Tao Te Ching).

An interesting parallel exists here between the Bible and Chinese sources of Tradition about the creation of the universe. In Lao Tzu's quote, the Tao is considered to be God and can be interpreted as: "In the beginning there was God and when God became self-aware, the whole was created. This whole was then divided into two main qualities (yin and yang). These two qualities are held together by ch'i – the immaterial breath that balances the two." (Source of Chinese Tradition). From this analysis of the Bible and Chinese Tradition we can see the roots of yin and yang, the backbone to Chinese philosophy and feng shui.

Yin and yang is a concept based on opposite polarities that move from one extreme to another in order to create a homeostasis or balance. This concept can clearly be seen in nature through the seasonal changes and time of day. The ancient Chinese astronomer evaluated the cosmos realizing there was continual change that followed a cyclical pattern. As you recall from chapter one, the ancient sages analyzed the big dipper's positions to determine the seasons. When the tail of Ursa Major pointed to the East it was spring. When it pointed to the South, it was summer. When it pointed to the West, it was fall, and when it pointed to the North, it was winter. They were able to determine the four directional points and cycle of the sun by utilizing an 8-foot pole and observing the shadows of the sun. The sunrise was to the east and sunset to the west. The longest shadow cast by the sun was to the north and the shortest to the south.

By tilting the pole to a right angle to the ground and observing the positions of the shadow, they determined the length of the year to be approximately 365.25 days.

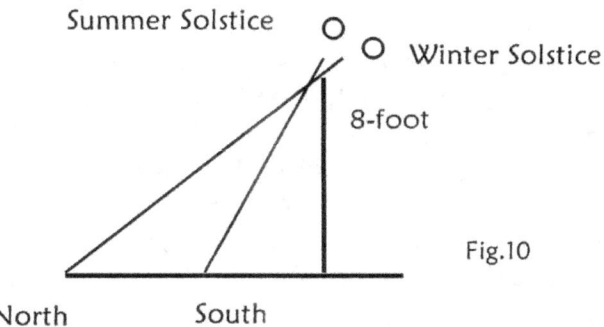

Fig.10

They continued the process further by dividing the year into twenty-four parts (agricultural cycle) and marking key points (spring equinox, summer solstice, autumn equinox, and winter solstice). They were able to come to these conclusions based on the sunrise position and big dipper. By using six concentric circles and dividing them into twenty-four parts they could record the daily shadow of the sun. The summer solstice represented the longest day and therefore the shortest shadow. The winter solstice represented the shortest day and therefore the longest shadow. Once they connected the points in the concentric circles, the sun chart looked like the Tai Chi symbol depicting the seasonal changes. The birth of spring (vernal equinox) slowly builds yang energy (waxing) until it meets its peak at the summer solstice. At this point yang energy begins to wane and yin energy begins to wax slowly to the autumn equinox and builds steadily until it reaches its peak at the winter solstice and the process begins again. This movement defines the waxing and waning of yin and yang energy.

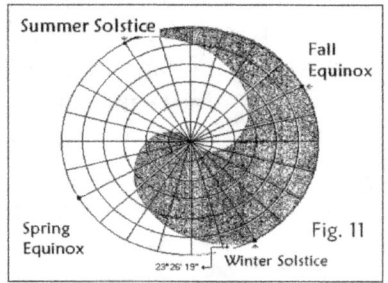

Fig. 11

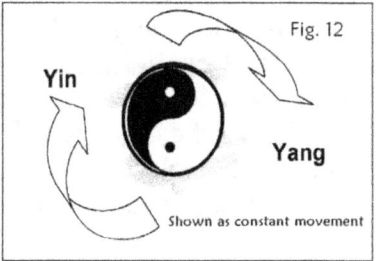

Fig. 12

Shown as constant movement

Yin and yang are two polar opposites that are always vying to dominate one another. However, total dominance is never permanent, as eventually the other will take its turn. They are the forces that drive the universe and depend on each other for harmony and balance. Like two fishes swimming to catch each other, as seen in the Tai Chi symbol, they depend on each other for the integrity of the whole. The outer circle represents "everything" while the inner black and white portions represent the interaction between the two forces (yin and yang). This continual interaction creates change in the universe representing the cycles of birth, growth, and decay. Ancient Taoist philosophers believe the interaction between these forces keeps the world spinning creating the universal life force energy or ch'i.

The yin component is the darker half where energy is being accumulated. It represents the earth, dark side of the mountain, female receptive qualities, the night, winter, cold, wetness, the moon, earth and metal, dark colors, passive behavior, death, softness, inside, downward movement, magnetism, right side of house, second floor of house, storage rooms, bathrooms, back of house, a valley, and rooms for relaxation. The yang component is the lighter half where energy is being expended in order to manifest something or take action. It represents the day, potential, electricity, light, heat, the sun, male dynamic energy, dry, spring and summer, wood and fire, space, light colors, activity, pointed shapes, mountain, left side of house, first floor of house, activity rooms, and work rooms.

Yin–Yang & The Human Body

Traditional Chinese Medicine embodies the principles of yin and yang to describe the body systems and the overall balance for physical and mental health. If we apply these principles to the body, the upper part of the body is considered yang while the lower part is considered yin. The skeletal system and exterior is yang while the interior is yin. The back is yang and the abdomen is yin. The internal organs are classified as yin and yang depending on the organ function. The yang organs are classified to the organs of the bowels (i.e.: gallbladder, stomach, large intestine, small intestine, urinary bladder and triple warmer). They are considered yang

Yin–Yang & The Five Elemental Energies

because their primary function is to transmit and digest food and water. These are considered action-oriented processes. The heart, liver, spleen and kidneys are considered yin because their primary function of preserving vital substance is a very stabilizing concept. In terms of the yin and yang between the five organs, the heart and lungs are yang because their physical location in the human body is higher than the liver, spleen, and kidney.

The balancing of yin and yang in the body is essential to thwart disease and achieve health. Looking at this from a practical standpoint, we can assess the activities of an individual and determine the harmony or disharmony that may exist. For example, a person who is very active, constantly working, starting new projects, etc. is always expending energy. Therefore, the yang component of their body is working over time and their yin energy is being squelched. Eventually the body will react by feeling exhausted and will need to rest in order to recharge the yin component and bring itself back into a state of balance. Traditional Chinese Medicine (TCM) believes that constant infractions to the body from the environment can create imbalances resulting in disease. These diseases are classified as being either yin in nature, (aversion to cold, loose stools, slow pulse, dark gloomy complexion, never thirsty, etc.), or yang in nature (fever, thirsty, constipation, rapid pulse) and is a direct result of one's immediate surroundings, activities, and food ingested.

One of the basic premises behind feng shui is to assess whether the environment has a balance between these polar opposites (yin and yang). If these forces are out of balance in the land and within the home, the occupants' personal yin and yang energy can be impacted. Below is a list of yin and yang external and internal environmental characteristics that have a direct impact on well-being.

Yang Environments:

- Hot climate
- Rooms or front of house facing East, Southeast, or South
- No vegetation to enfold the dwelling
- Highways or busy roads in close proximity to dwelling
- Parks or schools adjacent to dwelling during peak months and times
- Pointed objects directed at the dwelling
- Cities
- Airports and businesses within close proximity to dwelling

- Bright colors
- Vertical patterns, triangles, or pyramid shapes
- Spacious living quarters
- Elevated ceiling heights (over 10 feet)
- Hard furnishings
- Bright lighting
- Large windows
- Vertical blinds or no window treatment
- Mirrors and reflective surfaces
- Stone, tile, granite, and wood flooring without area rug

Yin Environments:

- Cold climate
- West, Northwest, and North directions
- Excess vegetation supporting the dwelling
- Quiet road
- Parks and schools out of season and time of day
- Curves and flowing shapes
- Rural areas
- Deep dark colors, muddy tones
- Upholstered furniture
- Soft lighting
- Smaller rooms
- Smaller windows
- Lower ceiling heights (below 10 feet)
- Heavier drapes and window treatment
- Carpets
- Rich textures and fabrics
- Lots of furnishings

Since the human body is constantly interacting with the surrounding environment, it behooves you to balance the yin and yang qualities. If you live in a city or around yang components such as a highway or business, then you need to balance that by designing your yard and internal space with more yin décor in order to counteract the overly yang external environment that will flood your home every time you open the front door. The same concept will apply to the overly yin external environment.

In that case you will need more yang components to bring about balance. The key is to harmonize the two qualities and work these energies synergistically with your own body and personality. Below is a list of yin and yang qualities. If you tend to be more yin, then increase the amount of yang in your space. If you tend to be more yang, then increase the amount of yin in your space.

<u>Yang Qualities:</u>

- Confident
- Enthusiastic
- Outgoing
- Strong
- Decisive
- Embrace change
- Finance
- Energetic
- Action oriented
- Intellectual
- Methodical
- Motivated
- Starts projects easily
- Slight physique
- Cardiovascular exercises
- Detail-oriented
- Science
- Math
- Aggression
- Analytical
- Speed

<u>Yin Qualities:</u>

- Sensitive
- Heavier Physique
- Creative
- Introspective
- Contemplative
- Grounded
- Slower Moving
- Nurturing
- Safety
- Yoga
- Meditation
- Philosophical
- Sadness
- Resting
- Intuitive
- Imaginative

When your body is exposed to too much of either polarity the qualities can be more dramatic as seen below.

Excessive Yang Qualities:

- Overly active
- Constantly on the run
- Exercise incessantly
- Not practical
- Future oriented
- Emotionless
- No attachments

Excessive Yin Qualities:

- Depressed
- Fatigued
- Weight issues
- Controlling demeanor
- Accumulate clutter
- Home body
- Emotional
- Stuck in the past

In addition to your external and internal environment, your diet plays a vital role in the yin and yang balance of your body. We are creatures of habit, and because of that, our diets may be rather routine and structured. On the following page is a list of yin and yang foods. Make an assessment of this list and decide where your diet tends to lean towards. The key is moderation and balance between the groups.

Yin Foods:
- Almonds
- Milk
- Alcohol
- Apples
- Banana
- Barley
- Honey
- Sugar
- Bean Sprouts
- Beer
- Oil
- Fruit juices
- Celery
- Clams
- Corn
- Refined foods
- Pineapple
- Shrimp
- Tomato
- Water

Yang Foods:
- Poultry
- Seafood
- Fish
- Cheese
- Beef
- Liver
- Peppers
- Eggs
- Coffee
- Peanut Butter
- Potato
- Turkey
- Walnuts
- Chocolate
- Butter

Neutral Foods:
- Bread
- Carrots
- Cherries
- Lean Meats
- Peaches
- Peas
- Plums
- Raisons
- Brown Rice
- White Rice

Once you assess your personality, environment, and diet you will have a better understanding of what category you fall into and can make adjustments for a more balanced life.

The Five Elements: A Sense of Harmony

The five elements (fire, earth, metal, water, wood) are the building blocks of the universe as a result of interactions between yin and yang. These elements from the Chinese perspective were active processes at work on the Material constituents of the universe, whereas the ancient Greek concepts of the four elements (fire, air, earth, water) were thought to be the actual constituents of the universe. According to James Legge in the book "The Great Plan," the descriptions of the five elements were as follows:

"Of the five elements, the first named water; the second, fire; the third, wood; the fourth, metal; and the fifth, earth. The nature of water is to soak and descend; of fire, to blaze and ascend; of wood, to be crooked and to be straight; of metal, to obey and to change; while the virtue of earth is seen in seed-sowing and ingathering. That which soaks and descends becomes salt; that which blazes and ascends becomes bitter; that which is crooked and straight becomes sour; that which obeys and changes becomes arid; and from seed-sowing and ingathering comes sweetness."

Each of these five basic elements was grouped with physical phenomena that influenced and created the five different sets of forces or powers. These forces followed the change of all things in the universe with a more sophisticated version of the yin and yang model of waxing and waning. The five elements represented stages or transformations within the yin and yang cycle whereby each element is said to flourish during its yang phase and decline in its yin phase. Therefore, the rising energy (yang) was given the wood ch'i representing the morning, spring season, and east direction. The peak and rising point of yang energy depicted the fire ch'i representing the summer season, noon, and south direction. As the energy slows down there is a building of the yin quality, the consolidation and pulling inward represented the metal ch'i, the autumn season, late afternoon, and west direction. The yin energy meets its peak and full contraction dissolves representing the water ch'i, midnight, winter season, and the north direction. The process begins again where the yang energy begins to resurge and the rebirth of spring and morning takes place.

The fifth element of earth was seen to be central to the other four elemental powers. It was originally seen as representing the ending of each season and beginning of the next. Hence, early fall may be so warm we refer to it as an "Indian Summer" and so forth. Eventually this elemental energy took its place between the fire ch'i and metal ch'i representing late summer/early autumn, early afternoon, and the center or ground point. The earth element was also considered to be the controller of the five elemental powers representing the soil ch'i energy and therefore the core basis from all things being accomplished. It was also seen as a pivotal point where the seasons were to revolve around.

The five elements were arranged in a systematic position that has the capacity to create or destroy one another giving rise to a new element. The first order is labeled as the birthing or enhancing phase. This is where each element is supportive to the new transformational energy.

Enhancing Transformation

Wood dynamically gives rise and fuels the fire ch'i energy. Hence, wood feeds the fire source. Fire enhances the earth energy by reaching its peak and dies leaving ash behind which becomes earth. The earth enhances the metal energy with its constant movement and contraction assisting in the formation of metal or ore. Hence, all ores originate from the earth. Metal enhances the water ch'i energy through contraction and the intense heat beneath the earth. This combination creates a liquid to flow like water. Water enhances or expands the wood ch'i, as it nourishes and refreshes all plants and trees, a wood source.

Diminishing Transformation

Just as the five forces of ch'i can support one another, they also can diminish one another. This occurs when an element is missing between fire and metal, metal and wood, wood and earth, earth and water, or water and fire. In the controlling or diminishing phase, the five elements work against one another. Fire destroys the metal, as its great heat will melt it into a liquid thus depleting its energy. Metal destroys the wood ch'i element due to its hard contracting force. Hence the metal axe cuts the wood. Wood diminishes the earth ch'i energy by its expanding movement breaking the earth. Hence roots uplift the earth and deplete its nutrients. Earth destroys the water ch'i by sucking it into its soil. Hence water saturating the soil becomes mud. Water depletes the fire ch'i, as it becomes vulnerable to its downward cooling energy. Hence water puts out the fire. We use this cycle in feng shui to balance excessive ch'i from an uncontrolled element.

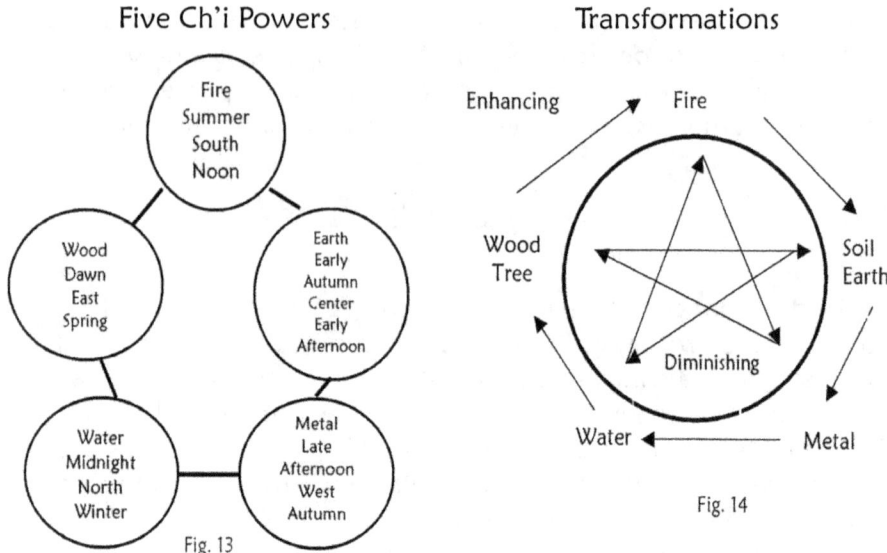

Fig. 13

Fig. 14

The Five Elements & The Human Body

The ancient Taoist physicians correlated the waxing and waning movement of the five ch'i elements in nature with the organ systems of the human body. The basic premise was how the influences of nature (i.e.: seasons, climate, time of day) affected the way man responded physically and emotionally to them. The phases of movement between these five elemental energies represent the pattern of human ch'i from one organ system to another following the enhancing cycle (i.e.: kidney-water, liver-wood, heart-fire, spleen-earth, and lung-metal). The second order of diminishing quality acts as a buffer to insure the birthing phase doesn't remain too long or too strong so balance in the systems is achieved. If a particular phase is overactive, then the phase is not being controlled properly and damage to the other phases or organs will ensue. As a result of this over activity, human ch'i becomes out of balance.

If we begin with the wood element we know in nature it represents growth, vitality, spring, birth, and the desire to achieve. The energy is expanding outward and in all directions. Therefore, it represents functions in the body that are self-regulating (i.e.: digestion, respiration, heart beat, metabolism).

Yin—Yang & The Five Elemental Energies

The liver is the associating organ since its primary function is to take minerals from food and convert them into energy for our muscles, tendons, and ligaments. The expanding ch'i associated with this element is connected to the emotion of anger demonstrated at the moment of birth with screams of discontent as we are taken from the comforts of our mother's womb.

The fire element in nature is when the yang energy is at its peak level. It represents the summer, heat, and upward forward movement. The corresponding functions in the body are those that reach their maximum level of activity and then begin to decline. The heart is the major organ representing this element, as heart rates can ascend, and at its maximum point begin to descend. From an emotional perspective, the fire element is the element of joy and represents a time in our life of pre-adolescents.

The earth element in nature is about harvest, abundance, and fertility. Earth energy moves horizontally, expanding and contracting, and is considered the stabilizer or center. These qualities correlate to the spleen, stomach, and pancreas with their location positioned in the center of the body or the core. The emotional component is one of a thoughtful or pensive state and equates to our adolescent years. This element represents the time of year where we pull ourselves inward and evaluate our resources for the colder months ahead.

The metal element represents the minerals within the earth. It is consolidating with an inward movement relating directly to the lungs and large intestines within the body. Emotionally, it depicts grief in our lives and equates to our adult years and a time to reap what we have sown.

The water element is one of the most profound elemental energies. This element is the sustainer of all forms of life on this planet. There is a strong correlation between this element and the human body. Water comprises seventy percent of the fluid that circulates within the body and is responsible for the nourishment of all cells. Water's downward and sideway movement corresponds to the kidneys and bladder systems.

Emotionally, water represents our fears and a time in our life of old age and accrued wisdom. On the following page you will find a chart that depicts the five elemental energies in a productive phase with their corresponding seasons, climate, body system, direction, and human emotion.

The Feel-Good Home :: Feng Shui and Taoism for Healthy Living

Wood	Fire	Earth	Metal	Water
Season: Spring	**Season:** Summer	**Season:** Late Summer	**Season:** Autumn	**Season:** Winter
Climate: Windy	**Climate:** Heat	**Climate:** Damp	**Climate:** Dry	**Climate:** Cold
Organ: Liver	**Organ:** Heart	**Organ:** Spleen	**Organ:** Lung	**Organ:** Kidney
Direction: East	**Direction:** South	**Direction:** Center	**Direction:** West	**Direction:** North
Taste: Sour	**Taste:** Bitter	**Taste:** Sweet	**Taste:** Pungent	**Taste:** Salty
Sense Organ: Eye	**Sense Organ:** Tongue	**Sense Organ:** Mouth	**Sense Organ:** Nose	**Sense Organ:** Ear
Tissue: Tendons	**Tissue:** Vessels	**Tissue:** Muscle	**Tissue:** Skin/Hair	**Tissue:** Bone
Emotion: Anger	**Emotion:** Joy	**Emotion:** Worry	**Emotion:** Grief	**Emotion:** Fear

The Five Elemental Foods

Traditional Chinese Medicine (TCM) attributes the five elemental energies to the flow of human ch'i and life. These elemental energies are susceptible to imbalances from the environment including ingested foods. By choosing a diet that can strengthen and replenish the elements that are deficient, the body can effectively return to a state of well-being. Listed below are foods that have the five elemental qualities.

<u>Water Foods:</u> Foods that fall within this element have a softening effect and promote moisture and relaxation. Those who have a slight physique, nervous, and have dry skin tend to benefit from this food type. Examples of some water foods include:

- Fish
- Shellfish
- Pork
- Beans
- Seaweed
- Soy sauce
- Miso
- Walnuts

Yin–Yang & The Five Elemental Energies

Wood Foods: Wood element foods have the ability to obstruct movement and can act as an astringent. People who tend to have erratic behavior will benefit from these foods. Examples of some wood foods include:

- Chicken
- Liver
- Wheat
- Sourdough
- Greens
- Citrus fruits
- Plums
- Yogurt
- Olives
- Vinegar
- Pineapple

Fire Foods: Fire foods have the ability to reduce heat and dry fluids. They most benefit people who are overweight, overheated, and aggressive in nature. Examples of fire foods include:

- Corn
- Peppers
- Celery
- Cayenne
- Coffee
- Tea
- Wine
- Alfalfa
- Asparagus
- Lamb
- Dandelion

Earth Foods: These elemental foods have the ability to slow down acute symptoms and neutralize toxins. People who are nervous, weak, and overly dry will benefit from earth foods. Examples of earth foods include:

- Dates
- Figs
- Grapes
- Peaches
- Carrots
- Cabbage
- Potato
- Squash
- Cherries
- Apple
- Watermelon
- Almonds

Metal Foods: These foods will promote circulation and most benefit people who are sluggish, lethargic, and cold. Examples of metal foods include:

- Tofu
- Rice
- Mint
- Anise
- Onions
- Turnips
- Rosemary
- Dill
- Radish
- Garlic
- Cloves
- Mustard
- Scallions
- Cinnamon
- Fennel

Birth Elements & Your Environment

In chapter two we learned about the three ch'i treasures and how they contribute to your personal ch'i. One specific component discussed was the planets positions at the moment of birth. The cosmic energy that emanates from the planets plays a role in your constitution and behavior. According to Western Astrology, the positions of the Sun, Moon, Rising Sign, and Horoscopic ID are the most powerful energies that affect you from a great distance. Due to this great distance, the effects are slow and gradual, albeit still important factors when it comes to your personal ch'i. From the Chinese viewpoint, the five elemental energies have a greater impact on your personal ch'i. This reasoning is based on the concept that you are an earth being that resides in environments that contain these five elemental energies. Since you are constantly interacting with your environment, then you are also interacting with those five elemental energies that will ultimately have an impact on you.

Like Western Astrology, Chinese Astrology has twelve zodiac signs. The characteristics between the Western signs (3 air, 3 water, 3 earth, 3 fire) and the 12-zodiac animals (rat, ox, tiger, rabbit, dragon, snake, horse, sheep, monkey, rooster, dog, pig) are similar in terms of their characteristics. The chart below simply demonstrates the parallel between the two zodiac systems.

Animal Year	Tropical Sign/Sun Based	Sidereal Sign/Stars Based
Rat	Sagittarius	Scorpio
Oxen	Capricorn	Sagittarius
Tiger	Aquarius	Capricorn
Rabbit, Cat	Pisces	Aquarius
Dragon	Aries	Pisces
Snake	Taurus	Aries
Horse	Gemini	Taurus
Sheep, Goat	Cancer	Gemini
Monkey	Leo	Cancer
Rooster	Virgo	Leo
Dog	Libra	Virgo
Pig	Scorpio	Libra

Personality & Psychological Patterns   Soul Nature

Fig.15
Chinese Astrology uses sidereal positions – Western Astrology uses Tropical

Yin–Yang & The Five Elemental Energies

One should bare in mind that the signs represent a modicum of the intricacies involved with both systems. Many people are familiar with this aspect of the astrology which is more commonly referred to as the horoscope. Unfortunately, it is more of a generalized perspective rather than a true read of the individual. Each system combines other variables in the computations along with an analysis of the interaction between these variables to personalize the type and quality of ch'i inhaled at the time of birth.

In feng shui practice, the goal is to balance the five elemental energies within a person's environment for health and harmony to ensue. Therefore, for the purpose of this discussion, we are referring to the Eastern astrology methodology. There are several elements to consider for a proper analysis including the self element (day pillar), birth animal (year pillar), hour animal (hour pillar), and month animal (month pillar). Also of importance is the predominant element within the chart. These four pillars (day, year, month, hour) contain specific information regarding the characteristics of the animal traits and balance of the elemental energies. Some of the energies will bode well for the individual, whereas others can cause obstacles and health challenges. The key behind interpreting a four pillars chart is to analyze how the daymaster (self element) interacts with the other elements of the chart. Furthermore, a close evaluation of the predominate and weaker elements is essential to determine what element(s) need to be incorporated into that persons environment in the form of objects, diet, or activities in order to obtain balance. To find your Chinese birth element, please refer to the chart on the following page. Understand this is only one aspect to the four pillars chart. A complete analysis is beyond the scope of this book. Please refer to the appendix for further information.

Chinese Birth Element Chart

Date	Element/Animal	Date	Element/Animal	Date	Element/Animal
2/19/1901	Metal Ox	1/27/1941	Metal Snake	2/5/1981	Metal Rooster
2/8/1902	Water Tiger	1/15/1942	Water Horse	1/25/1982	Water Dog
1/29/1903	Water Rabbit	2/5/1943	Water Sheep	2/13/1983	Water Pig
2/16/1904	Wood Dragon	1/25/1944	Wood Monkey	2/2/1984	Wood Rat
2/4/1905	Wood Snake	2/13/1945	Wood Rooster	2/20/1985	Wood Ox
1/25/1906	Fire Horse	2/2/1946	Fire Dog	2/9/1986	Fire Tiger
2/13/1907	Fire Sheep	1/22/1947	Fire Pig	1/29/1987	Fire Rabbit
2/2/1908	Earth Monkey	2/10/1948	Earth Rat	2/17/1988	Earth Dragon
1/22/1909	Earth Rooster	1/29/1949	Earth Ox	2/6/1989	Earth Snake
2/10/1910	Metal Dog	2/17/1950	Metal Tiger	1/27/1990	Metal Horse
1/30/1911	Metal Pig	2/6/1951	Metal Rabbit	2/15/1991	Metal Sheep
2/18/1912	Water Rat	1/27/1952	Water Dragon	2/4/1992	Water Monkey
2/6/1913	Water Ox	2/14/1953	Water Snake	1/23/1993	Water Rooster
1/26/1914	Wood Tiger	2/3/1954	Wood Horse	2/10/1994	Wood Dog
2/14/1915	Wood Rabbit	1/24/1955	Wood Sheep	1/31/1995	Wood Pig
2/3/1916	Fire Dragon	2/12/1956	Fire Monkey	2/19/1996	Fire Rat
1/23/1917	Fire Snake	1/31/1957	Fire Rooster	2/7/1997	Fire Ox
2/11/1918	Earth Horse	2/18/1958	Earth Dog	1/28/1998	Earth Tiger
1/2/1919	Earth Sheep	2/8/1959	Earth Pig	2/16/1999	Earth Rabbit
2/20/1920	Metal Monkey	1/28/1960	Metal Rat	2/5/2000	Metal Dragon
2/8/1921	Metal Rooster	2/15 1961	Metal Ox	1/24/2001	Metal Snake
1/28/1922	Water Dog	2/5/1962	Water Tiger	2/12/2002	Water Horse
2/16/1923	Water Pig	1/25/1963	Water Rabbit	2/1/2003	Water Sheep
2/5/1924	Wood Rat	2/13/1964	Wood Dragon	1/22/2004	Wood Monkey
1/25/1925	Wood Ox	2/2/1965	Wood Snake	2/9/2005	Wood Rooster
2/13/1926	Fire Tiger	1/21/1966	Fire Horse	1/29/2006	Fire Dog
2/2/1927	Fire Rabbit	2/9/1967	Fire Sheep	2/18/2007	Fire Pig
1/23/1928	Earth Dragon	1/30/1968	Earth Monkey	2/2/2008	Earth Rat
2/10/19/29	Earth Snake	2/17/1969	Earth Rooster	1/26/2009	Earth Ox
1/30/1930	Metal Horse	2/6/1970	Metal Dog	1/14/2010	Metal Tiger
2/17/1031	Metal Sheep	1/27/1971	Metal Pig	2/3/2011	Metal Rabbit
2/6/1932	Water Monkey	2/15/1972	Water Rat	1/23/2012	Water Dragon
1/26/1933	Water Rooster	2/3/1973	Water Ox	2/10/2013	Water Snake
2/14/1934	Wood Dog	1/23/1974	Wood Tiger	1/31/2014	Wood Horse
2/4/1935	Wood Pig	2/11/1975	Wood Rabbit	2/19/2015	Wood Sheep
1/24/1936	Fire Rat	1/31/1976	Fire Dragon	2/8/2016	Fire Monkey
2/11/1937	Fire Ox	2/18/1977	Fire Snake	1/28/2017	Fire Rooster
1/31/1938	Earth Tiger	2/7/1978	Earth Horse	2/16/2018	Earth Dog
2/19/1939	Earth Rabbit	1/28/1979	Earth Sheep	2/5/2019	Earth Pig
2/8/1940	Metal Dragon	2/16/1980	Metal Monkey	1/25/2020	Metal Rat

Fig.16

*To determine birth element: Person born between February 19, 1901 and February 7, 1902 is a Metal element and an Ox animal sign.

Yin–Yang & The Five Elemental Energies

The birth trigram is yet another factor that paints your personal ch'i and takes on a similar level of impact that the Western astrological system does. In other words, it has a slower more gradual impact on you. The birth trigram is based on the eight trigrams of the ba-gua and can be determined through the East/West Compass School computation. Below is the basic formula in determining your birth trigram with basic descriptions of the birth trigram numbers. We will use this formula later on to determine your personal ch'i directions in chapter seven.

Birth Trigram Calculation

1. In this calculation the year is based on the Chinese lunar calendar. Therefore, the start of the year is based on the mid-point between the winter solstice and vernal equinox (first day of winter and first day of spring respectively). The year begins then on or around February 4th. Thus, if you were born between January 1st and February 3rd, use the preceding year in your calculations. For example, if the birth date were January 8, 1989, you would not use 1989 for your calculation, but rather the year 1988.

2. Take your birth year and add together all the digits using a process of "Theosophical Reduction": 1961 1+9+6+1 = 17.

3. If the result is greater than 9, add the digits together again. 17 is greater than 9, so add its digits together; 1+7= 8.

4. If you are male, subtract the result from 11; if you are female add the result to 4. This is because males are yang and their essence or spirit is yin. So for males we subtract the result from 11: 8-11= 3. For females add the result to 4: 8+4=12.

5. If the result is greater than 9, add its digits together again.

Male = 3: No need to add. Female = 12: Needs calculation, so 1+2=3.

6. If the answer is 5, the trigram number is 8 for a male, or 2 for a female. The reasoning here is 5 does not have a trigram or direction on the ba-gua but it does have the earth element. It shares this element with the trigrams Kun (yin) and Gen (yang) depending on whether it is a male or female Ming gua. If this does not apply, then the birth trigram is the answer from the previous step, so in this case 3.

(*Note- This designation is based on Ancient Chinese Philosophy not Taoist).

Personality Descriptions of Trigram Numbers
(Based on Robert Sachs book: Nine Star Ki)

<u>1-Water Kan:</u> Represents the water trigram in the ba-gua. The ch'i personality of a 1-Kan trigram is strong to the core, a deep thinker, one who is developed socially, and listens intently. They can be an enigma, yet easily flow with the group when they need to. The water Kan energy is sensitive to their environment and finds circumstances can change easily in their life creating undo stress. The key for this trigram group is to flow like water with every situation. Since this trigram is related to the kidney and bladder systems, the 1- Kan water should pay close attention to the health of this area of their body. Good clean water and foods prepared with a balanced amount of salt (not over done) is important for maintaining these systems. It is also important the lower mid-section of the body (position of these organs) are kept warm. Exercises that include fluid like movements and incorporate stretching such as yoga or Tai Chi are excellent for the 1-Kan water trigram. Daily deep breathing meditations are also an excellent activity for 1-Kan water since they are prone to fears and anxiety.

<u>2-Earth Kun:</u> Represents the Mother Earth trigram in the ba-gua. The ch'i personality for 2-Kun is one of receptivity, dependability, mothering qualities, and kindness. The 2-Kun energy is devoted and hard working at whatever the task may be and enjoys being a part of a group rather than stand-alone. This trigram relates primarily to the abdomen and digestive system. The 2-Kun must therefore be aware of the foods they choose to eat. Since their nature is one of caring for others, they never find the time to care for themselves and, as a result, they tend to have poor diets leaving them susceptible to weight issues and blood sugar imbalances. The key for the 2-Kun is to take the time to care for themselves so they can be a better resource to others.

<u>3-Wood Zhen:</u> This trigram number represents the thunder energy in the ba-gua. The 3-Zhen energy is very dynamic, explosive, initiating, impetuous, and action oriented. They are quick thinkers, self-starters, visionaries, and intense when it comes to working. The body systems related to the 3-Zhen trigram are the feet, liver, and muscular system. The 3-Zhen individual benefits from a healthy level of exercise with a good amount of rest to counteract all their energy. They should avoid stimulates, dairy, and meats. Vegetables and fruits benefit the 3-Zhen person the most. Zhen trigram people benefit from yoga and meditative forms of exercise balanced with cardiovascular routines.

<u>4-Wood Xun:</u> This trigram represents the wind energy in the ba-gua. The 4-Xun energy has a keen independent and sensitive nature about them. They are very intelligent people who love to learn and strive to make it in life. They have an amazing ability to come up with new ideas, but find it hard to explain their point succinctly. Because of this, they are known to be impatient and can become frantic. The body systems associated with the 4-Xun is the gallbladder, thighs, and respiratory system. Their tendency is to suffer from lethargy or arthritic conditions depending upon the stress level in their life. It is best for the 4-Xun to partake in regular cardiovascular exercises such as jogging or swimming and to keep a diet high in green leafy vegetables and calcium rich foods.

<u>6-Metal Qian:</u> The Qian trigram is the most yang of all the trigrams in the ba-gua and represents the Creative or Heaven energy. The 6-Qian is very creative, active, initiating, and responsible type of energy. They are people who have strong ideals and are willing to stand up for what they believe. They are hard working individuals and achievers in life. However, at times they can be very self-critical and undiplomatic in their behavior. The ultimate purpose and meaning behind 6-Qian energy is peace, guidance, and truth. The head and lungs are the two main areas of the body connected to the 6-Qian ch'i. It is important relaxation is a part of the 6-Qian life, as undo stress created by their pride will lead to worry and tension. Inverted yoga positions are the best form of exercise for the 6-Qian, as the rich oxygenated blood flow will reach the lungs and head region.

<u>7-Metal Dui:</u> Represents the lake or marsh trigram in the ba-gua. The 7-Dui is a joyful, graceful, sensual, talkative, intuitive, and psychic. This ch'i energy is about accumulating the experiences of others and benefiting from it. As a result, the 7- metal may be viewed as being lazy. However, the 7-metal energy can be infectious, as they are optimistic and excellent communicators. They love the finer things in life and always manage to get it. The primary areas of the body that are related to this trigram element are the mouth, skin, colon, and lungs. These areas are prone to changes in climate, so protecting oneself from cold weather is important. Any type of rhythmic breathing exercises can be very helpful for the 7-metal along with a diet low in dairy and high in fruits.

<u>8-Earth Gen:</u> This trigram represents the still mountain energy in the ba-gua. The 8-Gen person has a simplistic contemplative inner knowledge about them. This energy is very slow and methodical with a keen sense of detail behind everything that is done. The 8-Gen is very competitive, yet exudes a sense of stability behind everything they do. They are very steadfast in their opinions and therefore have difficulties with change. The body parts associated with this trigram element are the fingers, hands, spleen, and stomach. Since the mountain represents a solid mass, it is important the 8-Gen participate in daily exercise and maintain a diet in complex carbohydrates and protein.

<u>9-Fire Li:</u> This trigram in the ba-gua represents the fire ch'i of the South. It is about expansion, clarity, charisma, passion, and brilliance. This is the public speaker that can hold the audience interest with their impressive appearance and charismatic personality. The 9-Li person is very trustworthy, loyal to others, and looks for support from friends and family. The 9-Li does not express their feelings very well and gives the impression all is well, even if it isn't, which can lead to anxiety and tension. The main body parts associated with this trigram element is the heart, eyes, and circulatory system. The 9-Li is vulnerable to cardiovascular diseases and therefore should maintain a vegetarian diet with some fish and practice a cardio-intensive type of yoga or Tai Chi.

The Five Element Energies in Décor

One of the main components to practicing the art and science of feng shui is to evaluate the elements within an environment and determine if they are balanced and supporting the occupant. On the following page are the descriptions of the five elemental energies and some practical design ideas. It is important that you evaluate your own space, especially in those rooms you tend to spend a great deal of time in (bedroom, kitchen, family room, office) and determine if the elements are balanced and adequately supporting you. Should you need to incorporate one or more elements into your life, you may do so through design, directions, diet, or the type of activities you engage in.

Wood Element:

Season: Spring
Direction: East (yang side) Southeast (yin side)
Time of Day: Sunrise
Ch'i: Uplifting and motivating
Activities: Physical exersion, writing, creativity, and brainstorming
Shapes: Columnar, tall, vertical patterns, stripes
Color: Green
Objects/Décor: Plants, wood furniture, floral prints, landscapes, flowers, pastels, columns, cotton fabrics, bamboo furniture

Fire Element:

Season: Summer
Direction: South
Time of Day: Noon
Ch'i: Expansive
Activities: Travel, outgoing, social, sales, public speaking, acting
Shapes: Diamond, pointed, pyramid, star, triangle
Color: Red hues
Object/Décor: Candles, animals, people images, leather, lighting, image of the sun or fire, feathers, wool, obelisk, fireplaces

Earth Element:

Season: Late Summer
Direction: Center, Northeast, Southwest
Time of Day: Late Afternoon
Ch'i: Grounding and settling
Activities: Meditation, yoga, or fire related activities
Shapes: Square, rectangular, low and flat surfaces
Color: Yellow, earth tones
Objects/Décor: Tile, brick, granite, check patterns, terra cotta, earthy landscapes, horizontal patterns, ceramic, lower ceiling (8 feet), some stones and crystals

Metal Element:

Season: Autumn
Direction: West, Northwest
Time of Day: Evening
Ch'i: Contracting, pulling inward
Activities: Mental processes, finance, gathering activities, communication
Shapes: Oval, circular, arches
Color: White, silver
Objects/Décor: All metals, round and oval patterns, natural quartz crystal (high paramagnetics), metal chimes, metal art or sculptures, arches in doorways or windows, coins, bowls, reflective items

Water Element:

Season: Winter
Direction: North
Time of Day: Midnight
Ch'i: Flowing
Activities: Sleeping, introspective, relaxing, swimming, conteplation
Shapes: Irregular, amorphous
Color: Black, dark blues
Objects/Décor: Indoor water features (fountains, aquarium), water scenes, glass, mirrors, outdoor water features (pond, lake, ocean, stream, pool), flowing drapes, gravel

 Now that you have an idea of these elemental qualities, evaluate your space and determine if one element is controlling it. By and large, you will feel uncomfortable in a room that is not balanced in the elements and polarities of yin and yang. Below is a list of how the elements can affect our attitude and behavior if they are out of balance.

Fire Element:

Excessive Fire: Anger, aggressive behavior, tendency for hyperactivity.
Depleted Fire: Feelings of unattachment.
Balanced Fire: Joyful and outgoing expression.

Earth Element:

Excessive Earth: Smothering energy, routine behavior, no risks.
Depleted Earth: Feelings of insecurity and safety issues.
Balanced Earth: A grounded and stable feeling in life.

Metal Element:

Excessive Metal: Constant mental activity and very talkative.
Depleted Metal: Ambiquity with no clear direction or communication.
Balanced Metal: Concise thought process and clear communication.

Water Element:

Excessive Water: Overly emotional and feelings of depression.
Depleted Water: Lack of emotion and disjointed life.
Balanced Water: Stable emotions and overall abundance in life.

Wood Element:

Excessive Wood: Self-oriented and rigid physically and emotionally.
Depleted Wood: Random behavior with no structure in life.
Balanced Wood: Empathetic qualities and helpful to others.

Combining Elemental Energies

When designing your space you can enhance or deplete an element using the two basic phases (enhancing and diminishing) of the five elements. Below are examples of how to utilize these phases within your space.

Enhancing Elements

Increase Fire: Place a fire element or a wood element since wood fuels the fire.
Increase Earth: Place an earth element or fire element (fire burns to leave behind ash or earth).

Increase Metal: Place a metal element or an earth element as earth spins and contracts to form the metal.

Increase Water: Place a water element or metal element as metal condenses and flows like water.

Increase Wood: Place a wood element or a water element as water nourishes and feeds the wood.

Diminishing/Reducing Cycle

The diminishing cycle is not necessarily negative even though it sounds as though it could be. Using this cycle can actually achieve harmony and balance while creating depth in designing a space.

Decreasing Fire: Add water to dimish the fire (water dowses the fire) or place an earth element to drain it. The constant burning of the fire to produce the ash of the earth will drain the fire.

Decrease Earth: Add the wood element to diminish it by uprooting the earth and absorbing its nurtrients. Add metal to drain the earth. The constant spinning and contraction to produce metal will drain the earth.

Decrease Metal: Add the fire element to diminish it (fire melts the metal) or add water to drain it. The constant condensing of metal to create water will drain the metal.

Decrease Water: Add the earth element to diminish it (earth absorbs water and dams it) or add the wood element to drain it. The constant feeding of the wood results in draining the water supply.

By balancing the two polarities of yin and yang energy and the five elemental powers through design of the external and internal environment, combined with the food you ingest (yin/yang/five elements), you can take control of your health creating balance and harmony within and around you.

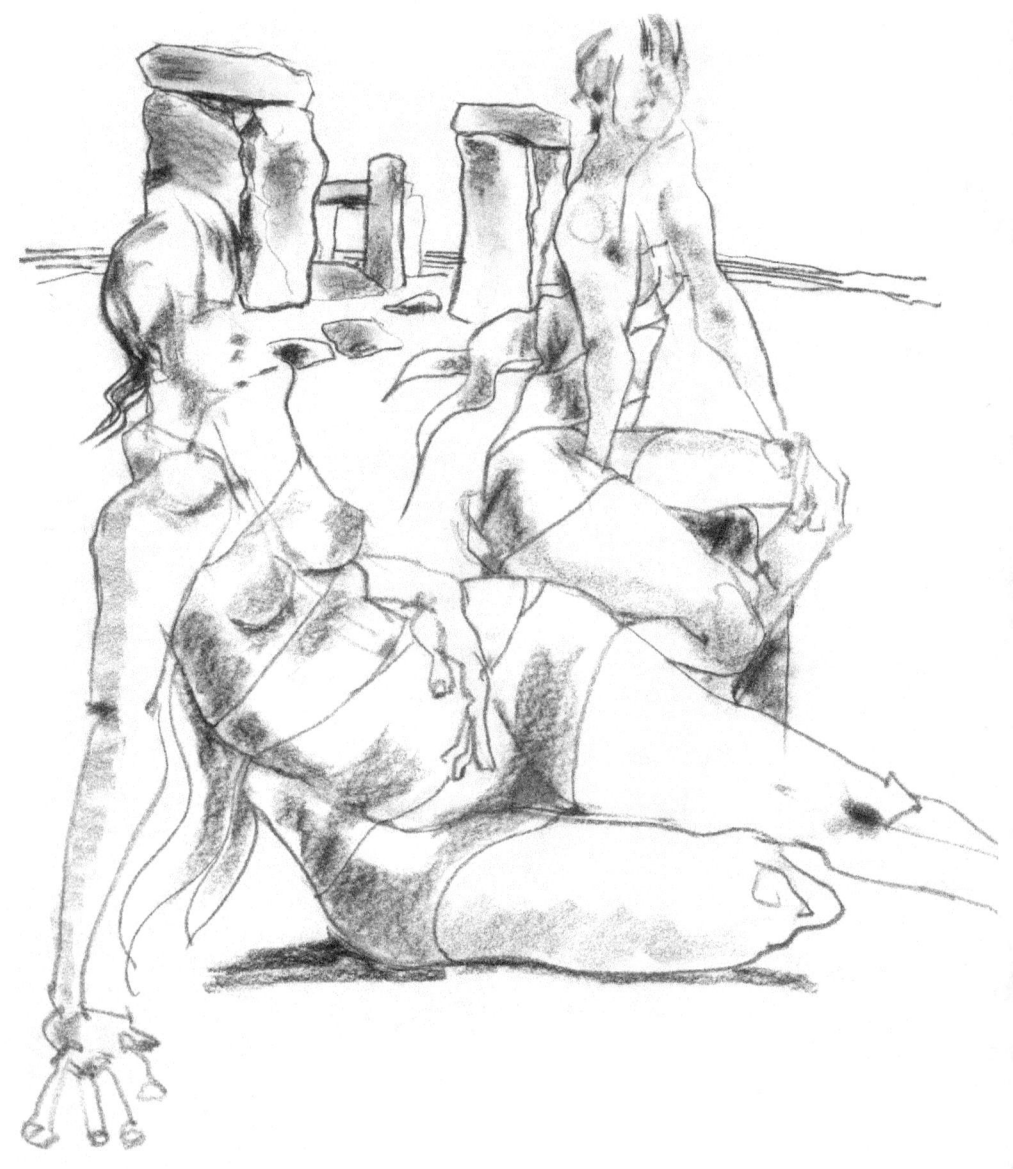

4
The Connection Between Earth Energies, Man-Made Energies & Disease

"Never, no never, did nature say one thing and wisdom say another."

Edmund Burke (1729-1797)

The earth can be thought of as a container that holds all matter together. It is an electromagnetic body comprised of many grids that are a result of interactions between various forces such as magnetism, electricity, light, color, heat, sound, and matter. These earth grids consist of lines referred to as "leys" that have been in existence since the formation of our planet.

Dr. Alfred Watkins rediscovered this ancient ley system in 1921 and referred to them as "straight tracks." He believed these tracks were used for various purposes including the building sites of many sacred places. Famous sites and Geographic locations such as Stone Henge, the Giza Pyramid, the Pentagon, Pyramids in China, many Native American reservation sites, Devil's Triangle near Bermuda, Antartica, Equator, the Tristan Stone, the Caves of Zimbabwe, Peruvian Monoliths, Sedona Arizona, and the Poles are some extraordinary places located on this intricate ley network system.

Along with Watkins rediscovery of the leys, a man by the name of Tom Graves discovered that underground water and "blind" streams (water coming to surface) followed these ley systems running beneath the ancient monuments and sacred places. Many of these water springs were considered holy because of their healing qualities. One place in particular is the Grotto at Lourdes France that is situated on a ley grid. Graves also discovered that many standing stones and stone circles were placed above these leys, especially in England. He considered these formations to be an ancient acupuncture system to balance the earth's natural energy system that otherwise can be disturbing for man, plants, and animals to live on. These standing stones and circles transmute the elevated earth energy vibrations emitted from underground streams, fissures, and faults to a slower rate that is more compatible for man.

The ancient Chinese sages were also aware of these elevated earth energies and avoided building houses on these stressful lines referred to as "Dragon Lines." This holds true for many ancient civilizations such as the Inca residents of Machu Picchu, high in the Andes, to the village in Orkney called Skara Brae. Today, man builds over these geopathic disturbances all the time and as a result we are seeing a connection between these energetic disturbances and disease.

Dr. Hartmann, a German physician, discovered a problematic grid formation with positive and negative energy waves. According to Dr. Hartmann, these grids consist of positive or negative parallel energy waves rising vertically from the ground to a height of 60-600 feet and can penetrate through buildings. The North-South lines appear approximately every six feet six inches and the East to West lines appear approximately every eight feet two inches. According to Dr. Hartmann, one of the most eminent experts in Geobiology and dowsing, more than 65% of diseases are due to anomalies and disturbances in the land. The most intense and problematic energies emanating from these lines are known as Hartmann Knots. Sleeping or working directly over a Hartmann knot resulted in diseases ranging from fatigue, insomnia, mood changes, joint disease, cardiac pathologies, and cancers. Dr. Hartmann was convinced after treating thousands of cancer patients over a period of 30 years, that cancer is a disease of location caused by geopathic stress.

During the same time frame, a Swiss physician by the name of Dr. Manfred Curry discovered another tighter grid pattern. He called this new network of lines the Curry Grid. These lines ran from Southeast to Northwest and Southwest to Northeast, with energy waves of approximately 6-8 feet. Where two negative lines crossed (curry crossing), disease of the joints and sleep disturbances occurred. Where two positive lines crossed, he found patients to have abnormal cell enlargement and, in some cases, led to cancerous growth.

Dr. Curry, a medical doctor and biochemist, ran studies of his own showing the connection between cancer and curry crossings. He surveyed many houses where cancer patients had previously lived. He did not know the patients or the specifics of their disease and by locating geopathic disturbances beneath their homes, specifically beneath their bed, could determine the nature of the patient's illness. The question comes to mind as to why these geopathic disturbances should cause health problems. To answer this question we need to know how and at what level the earth vibrates for health to ensue. Essentially, healthy earth energy vibrates at approximately 7.83Hz (cycles per second) and is considered to be identical to the range of human Alfa brain waves. Factors in the earth such as water radiation, leys, Hartmann or Curry grids, mineral deposits, geological faults, cosmic energy, magnetic fields, and man-made structures will distort the cycle of 7.83Hz to an elevated rate as high as 250Hz. This telluric energy (earth energy) will change with intensity according to the moon's phases. In particular, during periods of a full moon the radiation intensity is higher and will decrease as the moon wanes.

A United States scientist confirmed in the 1930's that humans (as well as animals) have less of a chance to fight bacteria, viruses, and parasites above 180Hz cycles. This occurs since the lymphatic system, which is responsible for transporting lymphocytes and antibodies, is affected by these geopathic disturbances. As a result, the immune system is weakened allowing the body to be overcome by bacteria and fungus making us prone to illness and disease, cancer being one of them. Furthermore, medical doctors have always found fungus and viruses in the blood of cancer patients making this a very interesting correlation.

Underground moving water is another source of potential geopathic earth energy. When water flows beneath the ground it will move along rock surfaces producing a series of overlapping spirals or water radiation. These spirals move in a clockwise and counterclockwise motion. The counterclockwise motion produces a healthy form of energy and creates a single spiral of wave energy that attracts like energy waves. The clockwise spiral forms a double spiral wave of unhealthy energy and this is magnified when two energy leys pass through an area of decaying material, better known as a polluted stream. This type of wave energy can penetrate vertically through cement and all floors in a high building or home. A person sleeping over an unhealthy spiral will feel fatigued and over time may experience other physical ailments since the body will read this wave of energy as a violent frequency causing extreme stress to body cells. In addition, it also has been noted that bacteria thrives in unhealthy spirals subjecting those living above them to higher positive ions in the air.

There are many indicators to look for in detecting geopathic disturbances. Paying close attention to your surrounding environment can give you clues to potential elevated earth energies. The list below includes how some geopathic indicators may present in your environment.

Outdoors:

- Bee hives – prefer unhealthy spiral
- Ants & insects migrate towards unhealthy spirals
- Abnormal growth on trees
- Uneven yard-sink holes
- Vegetation that never does well
- Cracks in foundation, sidewalk, or driveway
- Spiders
- Mice

Indoors:

- Cats tend to gravitate to unhealthy spirals
- Difficulty falling asleep
- Wake up regularly between 2 & 5 AM
- Feeling tired even after a good night sleep
- Nightmares or restless sleep
- Chronic health challenges
- Crying baby for prolonged periods of time
- Floor heated systems
- Cracks on walls, floors, ceilings, furniture
- Spiders, ants, bees, or mice that find their way in at the same point in the home

The aforementioned are signs of potential irregularities in the earth's telluric energy causing an increase in earth vibrational forces beyond 7.83 Hz cycles per second. These signs are a point of reference, however, to locate the actual point of unhealthy waves does require the expertise of dowsing.

Dowsing

Every culture dating back some 7000 years utilized a form of dowsing. The Egyptians, for example, used images of forked rods in artwork, as did the Chinese. Detecting problematic earth energy was a matter of practice, which later became an aspect of the practice of feng shui.

Essentially, ancient people viewed the world as nothing separate. They considered dowsing an innate knowledge used to ask for direction or guidance. The land was part of them. They were not walking on the land; the land was allowing them to walk on it.

Dowsing taps into this original way of knowing all things are connected. This connection is the portal for exchanging information between man and Mother Earth. Dowsing taps into the subconscious, which is connected to our conscious thinking. Essentially, our bodies carry a subconscious or intuitive knowing. We all have experienced, at one time or another, a feeling of unease in certain situations. Perhaps something as simple as taking a different route to work to find out later you avoid a big accident. That was your subconscious sending you a warning message.

Dowsing, in general terms, is tapping into this field of information, originating from the deep connection living beings share with Mother Earth and the universe. This is exactly how ancient people interpreted the energy fields of the earth. Today, dowsing is still used to determine geopathic fields and underground water. In addition, some medical practitioners specializing in energy medicine use dowsing for their patients.

In addition to traditional dowsing, there are modern geopathic detection devices, including geomantic field measurement devices, electromagnetic field detectors, radioactive detectors, and infrared thermography. The main point of this discussion is the relevance of earth energy and good health.

Electro-Stress & Disease

Studying the earth's telluric energy variations caused by underground streams, mineral deposits, leys, fissures, and faults have existed for thousands of years. The ancients learned to live with this intricate network system because they were more in tune with the land. Today, in this fast paced technology oriented 21st century, we have removed ourselves from nature and as a result become less aware of these energies that can impact the human body. In addition to the natural grid system that is part of this planet, our bodies are exposed to what is commonly referred to as "electro-stress." Electro-stress is very similar to geopathic stress but instead of being part of the earth's grid system, it is created by man-made structures. Although some diseases are the same due to this escalation of Hertz cycles, we also see a shift in new types of diseases. For example, in the 1950's diseases such as diphtheria, tuberculosis, influenza, polio, heart disease, and some cancers were prevalent. Today, diseases like chronic fatigue, arthritis, and cancers of the immune system (lymphomas, liver and intestinal) are more common. If we were to examine the major changes that have occurred within our immediate surroundings, it would have to be the explosion of electromagnetic fields. Just think about it for a moment; since the 1950's radio has increased ten thousand fold, TV more than a million fold, along with microwave communication, radar, and other sources of low frequency fields. That is an extraordinary increase in technology and yet such a short amount of time for the human body to adapt. The reality is it takes centuries for the body to acclimate to such massive environmental changes.

In order to understand the full impact that electro-stress has on the human body we need to understand what it is, and where it comes from. First off, electromagnetic fields are everywhere in our environment, including in nature and the planet itself. These fields are invisible to the human eye so we tend to disregard them. If we were able to visually see them, they would appear as a blanket of energy surrounding us.

To understand the complexities involved with electromagnetic pollution it is important to examine the electromagnetic spectrum. There are many different categories of energy that lies within this spectrum. Essentially, the higher you go on the spectrum, the wavelength becomes shorter, but the oscillations (cycles per second) or frequency becomes greater.

This defining point is the main characteristic between different EMF frequencies and how they interact with the human body. These electromagnetic waves travel at great speeds (speed of light) and are carried by particles called quanta. Quanta of higher frequency and shorter wavelengths carry more energy than a lower frequency with a longer wavelength. There are some electromagnetic waves that carry such an abundance of energy they are capable of breaking the bond between molecules. These types of electromagnetic waves are called ionizing radiation and are found in gamma rays given off by radioactive material, cosmic rays, and x-rays.

Man-made electromagnetic sources have a longer field wavelength and low frequency. These types of EMF sources are incapable of breaking molecular bonds and are classified as non-ionizing radiation. Some examples of these sources are radio-frequencies (RF), microwave frequencies, cell phones, microwave ovens, smoke detectors, MRI's, ultrasound, motion detectors, and alarm systems. Even though the frequency is insufficient to break the molecular bond, these EMF sources still pose a threat to living organisms, including us.

Electric Fields Verses Magnetic Fields

All frequencies along the electromagnetic spectrum have an electric field and magnetic field. Electric fields exist whenever a positive and negative electrical charge is present. The strength of the electric field is measured in volts per meter and present even if there is no current flowing. In other words, nothing needs to be connected to a circuit for an electrical field to be present. The strength of this electrical field directly corresponds to the voltage amount and distance from the wire source. Therefore, the closer to the source you are, the stronger the field. However, it will quickly diminish in strength as you move away from it. These fields are easily absorbed or shielded by walls, trees, buildings, and the ground. Therefore, when power lines are buried in the ground the electrical fields are barely detectable.

On the other hand, magnetic fields arise from the motion of electrical charges, or when the appliance or switch is turned on. These fields are measured in milliGauss (mG) and their strength is determined by the strength of the current source (appliance).

Similar to the electric fields, magnetic fields diminish in strength the greater the distance from the source. Unlike electric fields, these fields pass through walls, buildings, people, and the ground unhindered. Some materials such as concrete and steelwork can reduce the field strength, but not completely.

Static Fields Versus Time-Varying Fields

A static field represents an electrical current that flows in one direction, commonly referred to as a direct current (D/C). The earth's magnetic field operates under this flow pattern. The direct current (D/C) pattern is highly compatible with human cells.

Time-varying electromagnetic fields represent an electrical current that produces an alternating (A/C) current changing direction (reversing) at regular intervals (60 times per second). In most European countries, the electrical current changes direction 50 cycles per second or 50 HZ. North America has an electrical current set at 60 cycles per second and thus the electromagnetic field correspondence changes orientation 60 times every second. Unfortunately, research has shown if we had designed our electrical systems at a frequency of 200-300Hz, rather than the current 50-60 Hz, it would have been better for us. The best choice obviously would be direct current, but that simply is not feasible to handle the demand load.

If we put some things into perspective and compare man-made magnetic fields to those found in nature and the human body, we find that natural electrical and magnetic fields are relatively weak. For example, the earth's natural electromagnetic field is approximately half of a gauss (0.5G) or (0.00005T) Telsa unit. This is considered to be a massive number in comparison to the electromagnetic field of the human brain (0.0000000000000001T), which has an extremely weak field. Now, just to make some sense here, an extremely weak field to an electrician is measured at approximately 100G. This is a full billion times stronger than that of the human brain!

If we examine the electrical field component the scenario is quite similar. The human body, although electrical in nature, only puts forth a minute amount of electrical charge compared to even the smallest electrical circuits. Obviously, we can conclude that even the weakest man-made fields far surpass those found in the body.

Extremely Low Fields (ELF'S) & Exposure

In the electromagnetic spectrum two-thirds of the frequencies fall into the category of ELF'S, better known as Extremely Low Fields. These fields consist of power generating equipment, household appliances, and household wiring. Intermediate fields (IF) are found in computer screens, anti-theft devices, and security systems. Radio-frequencies fields (RF) are found in cell phone antennas and microwave ovens. What does all this mean? You live in a technology-based world that provides you with many conveniences and with those conveniences you compromise your health. Exposure to these magnetic fields influences the body just as they would to any other material made up of charged particles. These low frequency magnetic fields induce circulating currents within the body causing stimulation of nerves, muscles, and other biological processes. The key is to learn how to live mindfully in such an environment.

You can take measures to protect yourself from these electromagnetic sources by evaluating your immediate surroundings. The first area to begin your observation is in the bedroom. You spend nearly one-third of your life sleeping in your bed. During sleep your cells are 200 to 10,000 times more vulnerable to objects in your environment. With that being said, the bedroom should be the healthiest room in your home, but unfortunately when it comes to electro-stress problems, it is one of the worst. The main reason is the wiring configuration. The lights in ground floors run in the ceilings that are the floors to the bedrooms above. The cables for the second floor power supply run in the walls of the bedrooms, while the wiring for the upstairs lights run in the ceilings of these rooms. This type of configuration leaves the bedroom ensconced with wiring radiating 50Hz (Europe) and 60Hz (North America) continually.

This is not taking into consideration any outdoor infractions such as high-tension wires, transformers, or nearby factories that emit strong fields. Now, let's add to the mix modern day conveniences such as televisions, stereos, clock radios, phones, electric blankets, or water beds. These additional sources of electromagnetic fields bombard you during your most vulnerable time; sleep. Some modern-day conveniences are near the head while sleeping and can impact health. The worst offenders are clock radios and telephones because they contain transformers that emit powerful and persistent radiation.

Televisions are also problematic, as they emit very strong fields. When they are positioned in a family room the effects are less noticeable because the viewer is generally far enough away. However, in a bedroom many times the television is positioned close to the bed where the body can pick up the electromagnetic field. Secondly, most TV's have remote access and therefore the electrical fields remain live continuously.

Electric blankets and waterbeds are some of the worst culprits of electro-stress in a bedroom. These devices are designed to remain on the duration of the night, not to mention the actual contact with the body. There are yards of cable in these objects that emit a very dense EMF field. Even if you turn off the blanket prior to getting into bed, the loops of wire in the construction of these blankets allow for residual magnetic waves. At the very least, you should unplug them prior to getting into bed, but obviously the best solution is to avoid them altogether.

Another factor to be aware of is geopathic stress. If there are any unhealthy earth energies emanating into the bedroom, it will magnify any electromagnetic infractions. Dramatic improvement in health will occur just by clearing up the electro-stress and geopathic stressors in this room. This is easier said then done, but if you begin by eliminating the biggest culprits, such as electric blankets or waterbeds, that will be significant.

Replace the digital clock radio with a battery-operated clock. Move your cell phone or landline phone away from your nightstand. If you have a television in your bedroom, enclose it inside an armoire and disconnect the remote-control device. You can refine the field emissions from wiring configurations by installing a demand switch. These switches produce 4 volts of D/C (direct current) compatible with the human body. This device is ideal for circuits that feed the bedrooms, so the disturbing fields emitted by A/C will not occur.

Kitchen Electromagnetic Sources

The kitchen is another important room to analyze the EMF waves. Small appliances like blenders, can-openers, mixers, etc. will emit electromagnetic waves, but they are used with such a short duration of time that the resulting dose is negligible. One of the worst appliances for EMF's in the kitchen is the microwave oven. These ovens contain a device known as a magnetron that is capable of producing a very strong magnetic field consisting of short wave lengths at high frequencies. Remember, this type of frequency and wavelength is strong enough to break the molecular bond; therefore, it is important they are properly shielded and checked periodically. The key is to avoid using microwaves altogether. However, should this not be an option, at the very least avoid standing directly in front of them when in operation.

Electric Heating

Some households depend on electric for their heat source. By and large, this type of heat system emits high magnetic fields and trigger mostly during the night hours when we are most vulnerable. This occurs because electricity is more economical at that time period. When this heat source is provided as an under floor or ceiling heating system, it can be extremely problematic. The design is somewhat similar to that of an electric blanket where heat coils criss-cross the entire length of the floor or ceiling. These continuous electromagnetic emissions will constantly bombard the occupants.

Other Common Household Appliances

The use of personal computers exploded since the 1990s. What used to be a rare commodity is an everyday common appliance used for many hours during the day and evening. The screens are the most problematic component, emitting electrical and magnetic radiation with varying frequencies. This was especially true with older monitor screens. One type of frequency emitted is the (ELF) or extremely low frequency. This controls the screen display. Long hours in front of the computer screens can cause dry eye syndrome. This is most likely due to a build-up of static electrical charges on the skin and eyes, resulting in dust particles adhering to the eyeball. Research has shown that high numbers of cataracts were reported in patients below the age of thirty, especially when using older computer screens. Newer LCD monitors emit less radiation by mainly eliminating the spikes in the radiofrequency and electrostatic fields.

The key to protecting yourself from these emissions is to use a wireless keyboard and move at least three feet from the screen. The distance will drastically reduce the level of the emissions that you otherwise would receive. Placing quartz crystals, salt lamps, or salt candles near the screens will cleanse the wave emissions by reducing the frequency rate. They will also discharge negative ions into the air and counteract the positive ions released by the EMF particles.

Telephones & Lighting Sources

Telephones, although an obvious needed convenience, have drawbacks when it comes to field emissions. The powerful magnets embedded in the earpiece and microphone system release several hundred gauss frequencies. This is the reason why you feel tired or stressed after talking on the phone for long periods of time. The cell phone also emits electromagnetic fields, but these are fueled from a microwave source that pulsates from the antenna. Since the cell phone has direct contact with the head, the brain may absorb up to 60% of that energy. Studies, financed by the Swedish council for life work research, concluded that low levels of microwaves cause proteins to leak across the blood-brain barrier. Professor Salford and his team in 2003 linked the leakage of albumin (protein) across the blood brain barrier to serious brain damage. Obviously, the long-term effects are not yet proven, but it is possible these damaged neurons could repair themselves in time. Professor Salford goes on to report that these neurons would normally not become "senile" until people reach their 60's, however, they now do so in their 30's. Perhaps the most alarming concern is that cell phone users are younger and younger in age when cells are still multiplying and maturing and thus more vulnerable.

Lighting is another source of potential electromagnetic emissions within our environment. Some sources are better than others in terms of the magnetic field exposure levels. Incandescent light bulbs are one of the safest types of lighting sources for your home since they have very low emissions. Fluorescent lights, although more commonly found in office environments, can also be found in homes. This type of lighting source operates under a different premise than an incandescent bulb.

Fluorescents require a discharge to allow the inside of the tube to glow. Although their design allows for a longer life in comparison to the incandescent lighting, the EMF emissions are far greater. In addition to the higher field emissions, these bulbs discharge a high amount of positive ions into the environment. These positive ions account for poor air quality with a higher number of bacteria, fungus, and allergens leading to allergies and lethargy. Furthermore, the brain will respond to the flickering bulbs created by this type of lighting source by contracting and relaxing the muscles. This contraction and relaxation of the muscles deplete the magnesium supplies in the body. The result is a feeling of overall fatigue.

Full spectrum bulbs are yet another lighting source that closely resembles the brightness quality of natural sunlight. Although that is an attractive quality, this type of lighting is simply a fluorescent bulb with a higher frequency that eliminates the flickering element. Finally, there is the energy saving light bulb. These have become quite popular since they are able to conserve electricity. Unfortunately, with every positive feature there is a negative feature to account for. With this lighting source, the bulb is a miniature fluorescent tube, and therefore it emits a higher electromagnetic frequency. So, the bottom line is to stick with the incandescent bulb and natural light source.

Power Lines & Trains

Power lines emit some of the most powerful electromagnetic fields. These cables carry an excess of four hundred thousand volts or more. The humming and crackling sounds coming off these lines, especially when it rains, is the result of discharges into the atmosphere. Unfortunately, many homes and developments are built directly in the tracks of these cables. Living in close proximity to these cables compromises the health of the residents with minor complaints of headaches, allergies, nausea, and dizziness, to more severe ailments like cancer. Research has found that those who live within 165 feet of high-tension wires have a higher incidence of severe illness such as chronic fatigue, cancer, and blood disorders like leukemia. Some believe this is a result of their body cells absorbing the electrical radiation causing energy blockages in the body. When kinesiology or muscle testing was done on people who were within 330 feet of these high-tension wires, their muscles and joints became weak. Once they moved beyond 500 feet, their body systems grew stronger. Another problematic effect from high-tension wires is the high positive ions that are discharged in the air. This creates poor air quality and as a result allergies and fatigue can occur.

Radio waves and microwaves are another problematic source of external pollution that can compromise your health. These emissions occur from radio,

TV transmitting stations, and cell towers. The cumulative exposure from living in close proximity (0.6 of a mile) is when problems can occur. Those individuals having a lower tolerance level, such as children, the elderly, and the immunosuppressed (immune deficient) usually present with complaints first. The key is to avoid purchasing a home in close proximity to these problematic emissions. Trying to institute protective measures after the fact is extremely difficult and requires an expert dowser and feng shui consultant. Even so, when cell towers or high-tension wires are the offending agents, the situation is extremely difficult to remedy.

Satellite dishes are also problematic sources of emissions that have become a staple for so many homeowners. The parabolic dish focuses on incoming radio waves directed into a field horn. During the process, some of these waves bounce off the reflective parabolic dish while other frequencies are attracted towards the roof of the house. Those waves that bounce off the dish bombard whatever is in alignment with it. In other words, if your neighbor has a dish, and it points directly at your house, you can receive these indirect frequency waves. If the part of your home that is in direct alignment with the dish is within 17 feet, it may cause ailments such as headaches, low energy, and hyperactivity in children. The safest position for a satellite dish is 40 to 60 feet from the house with healthy vegetation surrounding it. Plants that will do best around a satellite dish are those that prefer acidic soil (Rhododendron, Azalea, Pieris), as the rebounding frequencies absorbed into the soil will cause it to be more acid base. To combat the scattered emissions from a neighbor's dish, simply plant high vegetation creating an absorbing barrier, or place a metal sheet in alignment with the dish as a deflective measure.

Trains & Assessing Risk Factors

Living behind a rail station is highly problematic in terms of the EMF waves emitted, not to mention the noise pollution factor. The magnetic fields that are discharged from the overhead supplies are comparable to those that are emitted from high-tension wires.

Needless to say, this is highly problematic and once again difficult to shield. The best advice in this case scenario is to move. If this is not an option, then create a barrier with trees such as Poplars or Gingos that have the capability of absorbing the emissions. They also have a tremendous capacity to counteract the positive ions discharged from the trains by releasing negative ions into the air. Planting vegetation will also act as a tortoise providing support and strength to the occupants. Placing metal chimes to the left side of the property will also aid in spinning sha ch'i away from the property.

Many electro-stress factors in our environment present health risks. When assessing these risk factors it is important to consider three main points. The first is the quantity of exposure. The second is the level of exposure. The third point is the threshold of the individual. This threshold is based largely on the age, size, and health of the person. Obviously, someone who is constantly bombarded by electromagnetic field emissions in his environment, internally or externally, will feel the effects over time versus someone who randomly is exposed to them. How our bodies react to these electromagnetic infractions varies, but many agree that an overload of positively charged ions affect the body's ability to remove toxins effectively. Basically, the blood leaves the heart with a negative (-) charge while toxins in the body have a positive (+) charge. The body is able to heal itself based on positive and negative electrical charges within the system. When the negative charged blood leaves the heart, positive charged toxins in the body are attracted to it. The blood will then assist the body in removal of these toxins. When we are exposed to electromagnetic fields, the level of positive ions discharged into the air escalates. As a result, the positive ions in the body can rise some 200-400 times. This creates an enormous imbalance between positive and negative charged electrical energy within the body. Unfortunately, the blood cannot function properly to assist in the removal of toxins. These toxins build and can lead to chronic ailments and disease. On the following page is a brief list of some health problems associated with electro-stress.

General Symptoms:	Nervous System:	Heart/Circulation Disturbances
o Headaches o Weakness o Fatigue o Dizziness o Bloated feeling o Disturbed sleep o Nausea	o Loss of concentration o Tendency to perspire o Slight tremor of fingers o Low blood pressure	o Elevated heart rate o EKG changes o Enlarged heart muscle

Protective Measures

The most obvious form of protection is to avoid the exposure as best you can. However, the reality is electromagnetic fields are a part of our world. We have a choice to either deal with them intelligently or to ignore them. Below is a list of self-help measures to protect against EMF infractions.

- Keep your distance from the source; EMF's dramatically decline with distance
- Remove the source whenever possible, especially in bedrooms
- Select equipment with low emissions
- Make sure equipment is in good working order
- Disconnect the remote control from televisions
- Unplug appliances not in use, especially computers
- Use demand switches when possible for bedroom circuits
- Make sure cables are shielded
- Have an electrician test all outlets and circuits for any leakage
- Be aware of outside environment prior to purchasing a home for any EMF sources
- Bring in plants that purify such as Rubber, Peace Lilies, Dracaena, Cactus, and Ferns
- Use salt candles or salt lamps to increase the amount of negative ions circulating in the air
- Minimize the amount of synthetics within the home, as they produce a static charge

- Do not use fluorescent lighting of any kind
- Keep cell phone use to a minimum
- Do not use a lap top computer on your lap
- Eat a diet rich in antioxidants, fruits, vegetables, and supplements
- Obtain protective devices designed to be worn or carried to increase the body's ability to resist the stressful effects of external fields (see appendix)

Feng shui is all about manipulating energy to benefit your life. The external and internal components of your environment are essential in the analysis. A thorough assessment of all electro-stress agents should be conducted with remedies instituted to optimize the environment for healthy living.

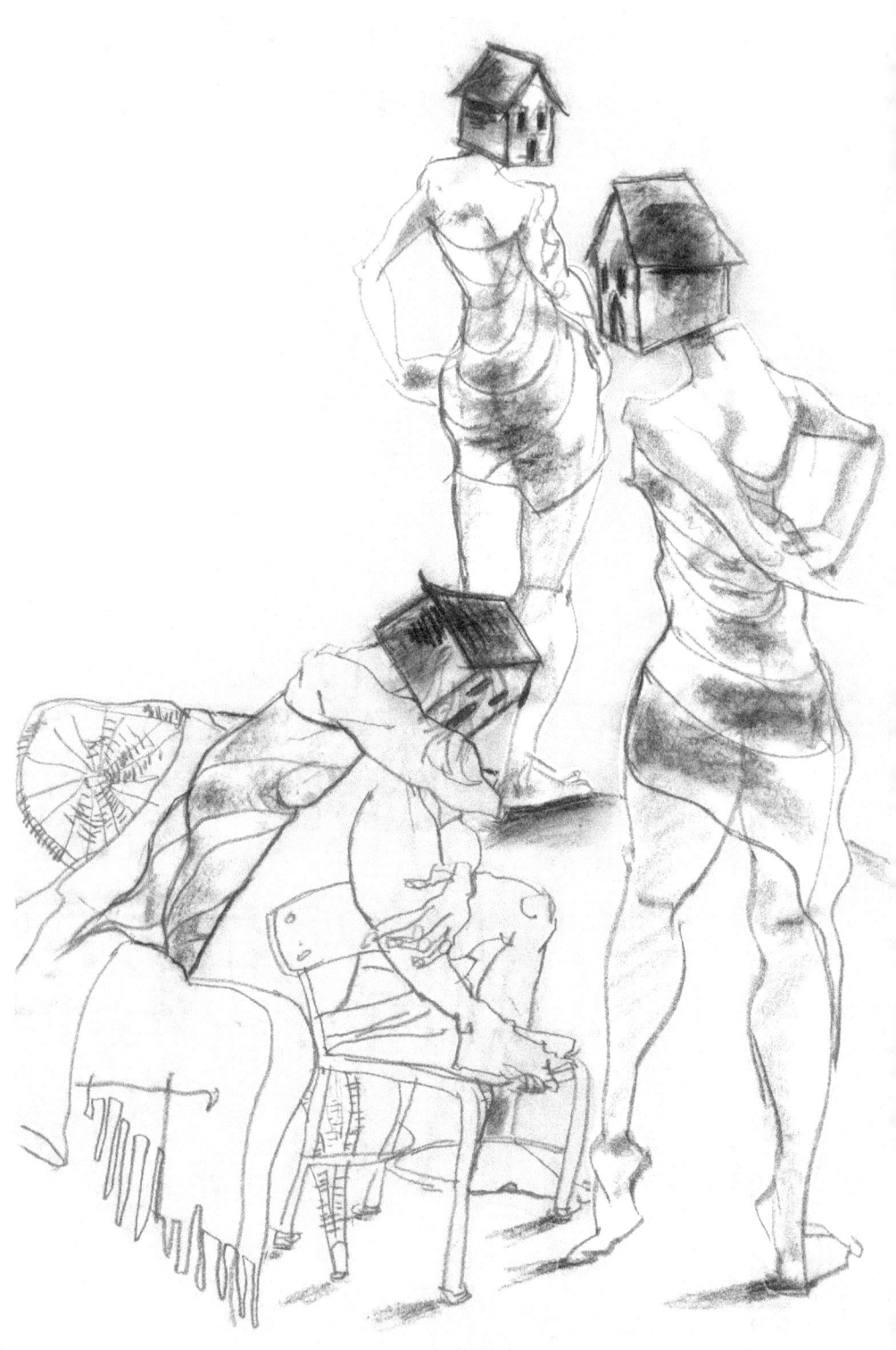

5
The Human Living Space

"Buildings, too, are children of Earth and Sun."

Frank Lloyd Wright

Since the beginning of time man has searched for a protective site to call home. In the past, this search involved the practice of Geomancy (study of the land) to locate the most auspicious site to settle. We know the ancient sages of China, Arabia, Europe, and North America followed these practices. For example, in ancient China the Emperor and high officials would consult the feng shui master to survey the land for the building of temples, palaces, and cities. The initial assessment always included a close analysis of the soil and terrain. The feng shui master, with his porter, would evaluate the soil by rolling it between their fingers to determine the texture. If it was supple and rich in color, it indicated the ch'i was very auspicious and able to sustain life. Tasting the soil for acidity (bitter) or alkalinity (bland) was part of the process to determine if the soil's mineral content was balanced. The feng shui master and his porter would then examine the terrain for any outcroppings, depressions, or dramatic land features. Any unusual anomalies were signs that a disproportionate amount of ch'i was circulating beneath the earth resulting in powerful earth energies (leys or geopathic stress). Depressions or sinkholes were also indicators that underground water was present and therefore problematic to build on.

Evaluation of the vegetation, its shape, color, and proliferation were additional determining factors of the strength and vitality level of ch'i within the land. Obviously, if the vegetation were not vibrant and thriving, then human life would also lack these qualities. The sounds and smells that emanated from the land determined the quality of the ch'i as a result of the continuous cycle of birth, growth, decay, and rebirth. Any odors that were pungent represented decayed ch'i and were unable to sustain healthy and prosperous living.

The heavenly directional influences, climate, and land topography were other mitigating factors to determine if a location was appropriate to build on. The land topography should mimic the four celestial animals creating an armchair effect to offer support, a view, and prosperity. The high mountain to the back or north represented the tortoise and provided support, tenacity, and longevity for the building and occupants. High undulating hills to the left or east represented the green dragon, and lower wider hills to the west or right, represented the white tiger. Both land formations provided support to the sides of the building holding vital ch'i in on the dragon side and dispersing stagnant ch'i on the tiger side. Finally, an open view to the south or front with a lower hill or footstool afar represented the spreading wings of the phoenix. This furnished the site with incoming ch'i to feed the building and occupants. These land observations became part of a verbal report to the Emperor for a final location to build the palace.

Today, modern day feng shui practitioners carry out a similar process in determining an auspicious site for building a dwelling. The type of soil base is still an important factor to consider. Interestingly enough, as early as 1929, Russian engineer George Lakhovsky discovered how certain soil bases (water filled clay) conduct EMF radiation. This type of soil is unable to fully absorb the suns radiation and, as a result, a secondary radiation is emitted into the environment disrupting the oscillatory equilibrium of human cells. Once this happens, the cell can no longer oscillate according to the natural frequency, and the ultimate result is break down in health and manifestation of disease. In his research, Lakhovsky determined that soils permeable to the cosmic and solar rays such as sand, sandstone, gravel, limestone, etc. were able to absorb external radiation to a great depth. Therefore, they did not formulate the secondary radiation that he found to be a contributing factor of illness and disease, especially cancers. In addition to noting the type of soil base, determining the acidity or alkalinity is important. Obviously, in feng shui we are always looking to balance energies, objects, materials, and other factors within the environment. Therefore, if the soil is overly acidic it would affect the equilibrium of the land.

An easy way to determine if the soil is acidic is to assess the type of surrounding vegetation. Many times when a property consistently presents with brown withered patches, very few animals frolicking about, an abundance of pines, rhododendron, spruces or hemlocks, it is indicative of high acid levels. By and large, external EMF sources such as cell towers and high-tension wires are responsible for such high acid levels making this type of property a poor choice to build or purchase a home on.

There are many other qualities to take into account regarding the vegetation when assessing a property. The type of species, height, number, and the proximity to the building, all play a factor in whether a property is considered auspicious. Trees positioned too closely to the dwelling will interfere with the foundation, windows, roof, and sidewalks. Any infringements on the structure will reflect in the health of the occupants. Removal or strategic repositioning of trees is imperative to meet the healthy environment specifications. Certain types of plant species will also determine the quality of ch'i that circulates the property. Weeping willows bring ch'i flow downward, while rose bushes, cactus, holly or bougainvillea represent a threatening or attacking ch'i because of their thorny nature. This is especially true when planted in close proximity to pathways, doorways, and windows. It is best then to plant this type of vegetation only if there is enough room for growth without infringing on these areas of the home. By and large, a property with a variation of plant species that maintain vitality throughout seasons translates into health, longevity, and growth for the occupants.

One of the most important land assessments is the protective features, or four celestial animals. Protection translates into safety, and when you feel safe, your mind and body can relax. These attributes in life certainly outweigh having a lot of money. Property that is well protected can be guarded by natural or artificial formations in the environment that will cradle the back, sides, and front of the dwelling. In rural areas, the four protectors (Dragon, Tiger, Tortoise & Phoenix) can usually be found within nature. The dragon side, to the right when looking at the dwelling, should be higher ground with trees; the tiger side, to the left when looking at the dwelling, should be lower trees, bushes, or rock formations; the phoenix to the front should be wide open with mountain ranges afar to cushion incoming forces, yet not to obstruct the view. The back of the lot should be the highest feature providing overall stability and support for the occupants.

By and large, most dwellings are located in an urban setting and therefore feng shui practitioners will associate the traditional landforms to surrounding buildings, roadways, vegetation, and other dwellings. For example, the green dragon formation could present as a building, large home, or high tree, preferably in a green color, and be placed to the right of the structure when viewing from a front perspective. The white tiger may take on the presence of a lower building, white fence or lower shrubbery to the left side of the structure when viewed from the front perspective. The phoenix might be a wide-open front yard, wide-street, or some open ground between it and the next facade. Finally, the tortoise should present as a larger home, building, trees, or fence behind the dwelling to hold in the circulating ch'i, while offering support. Keep in mind, the tortoise feature should not be too close in proximity to the dwelling; otherwise, instead of providing stability and protection, it will take on a suppressive feeling and squelch the ch'i. Having good Form School topography is essentially ninety percent of the feng shui formula for stability and good health.

Lot Shapes & Positions

There is much to consider when choosing a site to build on or when purchasing an existing property. The dynamics involved have a direct influence on your health and livelihood. If we begin by analyzing the symmetry of a lot, the square or rectangular shape is considered the most auspicious. These shapes encompass the entire ba-gua and offer a sense of balance on a conscious and subconscious level. Unfortunately, most lot dimensions are irregular because they are cut based on the land topography. Local housing developments or city housing are more likely to be a square or rectangle since they operate under parallel street designs.

In a traditional feng shui lot analysis, the property is divided into three segments. These three segments represent the family generations and their inheritance. The front one-third of the lot represents the parents or first generation, the middle one-third represents the children or second generation, and the last one-third represents the grandchildren or third generation. This concept was established since dwellings remained in

The Human Living Space

a family for generations. Essentially, a lot that is narrow in the front and progressively increasing in size to the rear was indicative of the first generation (parents) making great sacrifices with little benefits. In this lot scenario, the children and grandchildren benefit from the parent's efforts. The trapezoid shape makes it difficult for the ch'i to enter, but once it does enter it can grow and expand towards the back. It is best not to purchase a trapezoid lot since it will require great efforts with little reward. To remedy this type of lot, place spotlights on either side of the front yard along with any other ch'i activating devices such as bright colored landscaping, chimes, a water feature, or a bird feeder. The idea is to entice the ch'i to enter and modulate freely.

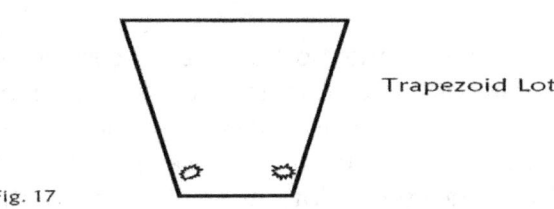

Fig. 17   Trapezoid Lot

A lot that is the opposite of the aforementioned is the inverted trapezoid property. This lot is wide in the front and tapers off to the rear. The first generation (parents) consumes the wealth leaving nothing for future generations. In this scenario, ch'i rushes in and is plentiful but dissipates quickly taking with it the prosperity for future occupants. The key to bringing some balance back to this lot shape is to install a fence or plant shrubbery to trap the good ch'i once it has flowed in. Balancing the lot in this way creates support and closure to the rear of the property.

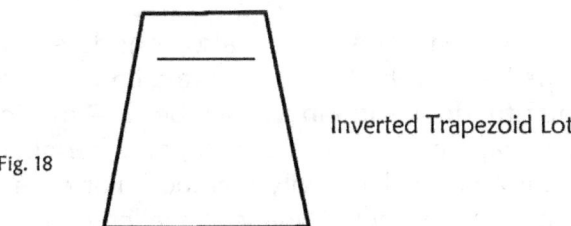

Fig. 18   Inverted Trapezoid Lot

Lots that have irregular sides mimicking a corrugated texture are indicative of unstable family assets. In such a scenario, it is best to plant a row of bushes on both sides of the property, with higher vegetation on the dragon side. This will give the illusion of smooth edging and stabilize the assets for the occupants.

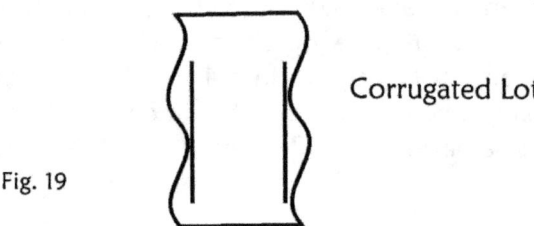

Fig. 19

Corrugated Lot

The triangular lots are the most problematic and should be avoided altogether. The angles that are created from this lot shape throw (sha) ch'i to neighboring homes. This is considered inauspicious in feng shui, as you never want to launch an attack against someone else. The best attempt to balance such a lot is to cut the apex of the triangle by installing a fence or trellis to this sector. Positioning a lamppost on either side of the front yard will soften the points and strengthen the otherwise weak corners.

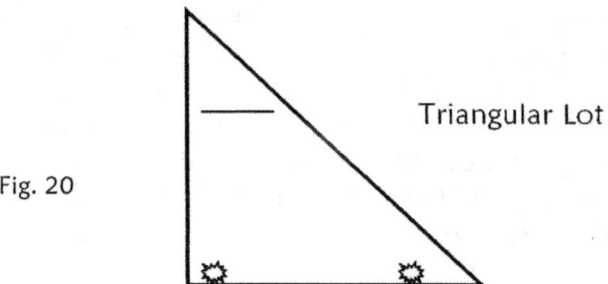

Fig. 20

Triangular Lot

An L-shaped or meat cleaver lot is also considered inauspicious. According to the ba-gua, the land has certain corners associated with our daily living situations and family members. A missing section caused by the L-shape can result in challenges in certain aspects of the occupant's life or a particular family member. For example, a missing left quadrant indicates potential financial challenges and difficulties for the eldest female.

The Human Living Space

If the L-shape lot is missing the far right quadrant, then relationships can be challenging for the occupants, along with potential health challenges for the mother. There are two options in creating a balanced lot (square). The first option is to plant hedging or install a fence to square off the lot. The remaining section can be treated as a separate alcove for gardening or perhaps a private Zen area. The second option is to generate activity closer to the missing quadrant with lighting, a bird feeder, a water feature, chimes, gazing ball or anything that will create movement. Use a symbolic object relating to the missing sector to gain back the otherwise depleted ch'i from this irregular shape.

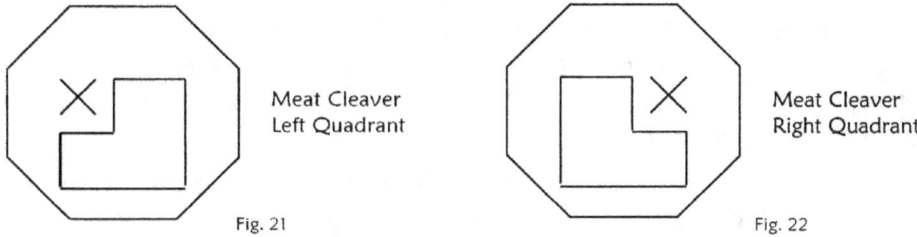

Meat Cleaver Left Quadrant

Fig. 21

Meat Cleaver Right Quadrant

Fig. 22

Lots that are positioned on top of a hill or at a low point, in comparison to other lots, are considered inauspicious. When a dwelling is positioned at the highest point it is known as "sitting on the back of the dragon." This is a rather unsteady position exposing the occupants to high winds, excessive ch'i, and overwhelming energy. The occupants are in a vulnerable position and as a result are unable to accumulate beneficial ch'i. Opportunities will literally move in and out of their life making it difficult to experience prosperity. Furthermore, the constant movement of wind will cause the occupants to feel unstable, restless, and irritable. Trying to shield these homes with trees against the harsh winds is a minor solution at best. Likewise, it is also inauspicious to live on upper floors of a high-rise building. Again, this simulates living on top of the dragon's back exposing the occupant to destructive energy.

On the other end of the extreme, is the lot that is situated at the lowest point in comparison to other lots. This position attracts overly yin ch'i and negative energy. The occupants will feel vulnerable from the overabundance of yin ch'i compromising their physical and emotional state. In addition, the neighbors positioned at a higher point will in essence have a foothold over the occupants beneath them. This leads to stress and compromised health. Properties in this scenario are very difficult to remedy and should be avoided entirely. If you have no other alternative, then energetically the property should be designed more towards the yang polarity. This can be achieved by projecting spotlights upward towards the roof of the house, bright colored flowers, upward vegetation (cypress, arborvitaes), stone circle formations using sacred shapes (circle, pyramid), reflective stones (mica, granite), water features, metal chimes, and reflective objects. In order to establish harmony between neighbors, simply place a soothing chime or water feature between the properties. This will infuse any negative energy with a peaceful sound vibration.

The incline or slope lot presents an interesting perspective. Many view a steep incline as an auspicious position for a home. However, a steep front yard presents an overall challenge for the occupant. It is very difficult for ch'i to navigate upward and as a result the occupants will experience difficulties in obtaining opportunities that may come their way. It presents as a constant uphill battle to achieve their goals mimicking the effort it takes to drive up or walk up to the entrance. A solution to this case scenario is to create tiered landscaping allowing the eye to gradually ascend the property. Installing spotlights at the down slope, and projecting the light towards the roof, will guide energy upward giving the illusion of a balanced lot.

The opposite of the steep incline lot is the flat terrain. When feng shui was developed thousands of years ago in China, land analysis was mainly considered for agricultural purposes. A flat terrain was considered inauspicious since ample drainage for crop growth was problematic. Classical feng shui doctrines adopted this theory and recommended dwellings be built on sloping land. However, the reality is most neighborhoods are built on a flat terrain and in essence provides a sense of stability and a solid foundation. These are two major components for healthy living.

Properties positioned in close proximity to a large body of water like an ocean are problematic. Although water is a very propitious element in feng shui, the ocean is unpredictable and can be ferocious. The constant surge and pounding of the ocean's surf directed to the mouth of the property is overbearing and can result in behavior that is out of control. Ocean front properties command top dollar in real estate and therefore make good investments, but from a feng shui health perspective, it's best to choose a lot with a calmer waterway. Strategically placing large rocks in the front of the property to create a barrier wall is a helpful shielding remedy against the otherwise threatening ocean.

Purchasing a lot that is sandwiched between two larger buildings or substantially larger homes presents with difficulties for the occupants. These larger structures dominate the smaller structure leaving the occupants feeling suppressed and in despair. It is as if someone is constantly standing over you, suffocating your aura and energy field. Many times the occupants will suffer from back pain, as symbolically they are trying to hold up these larger structures from collapsing onto their home. It is best not to purchase a home with this case scenario, but if this should be the case, placing a convex mirror on the smaller home directed toward the larger structure will give the illusion these structures are smaller. Planting higher columnar shaped hedging, and installing upward spotlighting to the smaller structure, will give the eye a visual balance to the property.

Road Positions & Signs

In ancient China waterways were the source of transportation for materials, people, and ch'i. Today, although waterways are still utilized, the intricate network of roadways have become the primary source of transportation. In feng shui these roadways are referred to as the purveyors of ch'i. The road design and flow pattern will determine if the ch'i feeding the property or home is healthy (sheng) ch'i or unhealthy (sha) ch'i.

There are many scenarios to consider when it comes to roadways and the type of ch'i that is associated with them. One of the most common placements for lots with homes is a straight road. This only presents as an issue if the road is heavily traveled, since the ch'i is transmuted by factors such as noise pollution, EMF's, carbon monoxide emitted from the cars, and overall chaos created by fast moving vehicles. This translates into a stressful environment causing fatigue and possible illness. If the road is less traveled, then a peaceful feeling will ensue for the surrounding residents.

Lots and homes positioned at the head of a T-junction or Y-junction creates a tumbling torrent ch'i directed at the mouth or entering point of the property and home. Here the ch'i will continue in motion until something in its path absorbs it. Unfortunately, many times this is the entrance to the home that now envelops the occupants with destructive forces. This position has a greater impact on the human body when the front door or bedroom is aligned to the T or Y-junction. The headlights from the oncoming vehicles, or better known as "tiger eyes," penetrate the home leaving the occupants with an uneasy feeling. Eventually, this road position in relation to the dwelling can take its toll on the immune system. In this scenario, the body is in a constant "fight or flight" mode and causes a release of adrenaline and other hormones. This is a potential precursor to fatigue and illness. The best solution is to avoid purchasing properties located on a T or Y-junction. However, if you are already in a property like this, then installing deflective and absorbing remedies is essential. Designing a curved land formation with strong vegetation and including reflective landscape accents with mica, granite, or exotic colorful glass, will effectively absorb and deflect problematic ch'i. Hanging a metal chime to the left side of the property will also assist the ch'i to spin and move around the property, rather than hitting the front door directly.

Cul-de-sacs, dead-ends, and corner lots seem to attract many homebuyers, especially those with children. Unfortunately, from the feng shui perspective, these road positions are highly problematic. The dead-end road is the worst scenario, as it creates a straight path for the ch'i to run directly to the lot or home positioned at the end point. The narrow path causes the ch'i to stagnate with charged pollutants from oncoming vehicles in the neighborhood, or the "wrong turn" driver.

The Human Living Space

As a result, this ch'i enters the home bringing with it pollutants, stagnation, and overall sha energy, a prescription for unhealthy living. The cul-de-sac operates pretty much under the same premise, but the circular configuration allows the ch'i to expand further and is dispersed between several homes positioned around the bend. If the cul-de-sac is designed with an island containing rich vegetation and large landscape rocks, most of the sha ch'i is absorbed prior to entering the property, and therefore is more auspicious then a cul-de-sac without the island. The best remedies for these road configurations are absorbing and deflecting modalities. Using landscaping, rocks, reflective objects, and chimes will all help mitigate the polluted ch'i source. Once again, the best solution is to avoid these property locations entirely.

The corner lot presents as a larger piece of property and therefore very attractive to perspective buyers. However, these lots are generally positioned disproportionately leaving the occupants with a feeling of being unbalanced. This type of lot position supports the home with roadways in two directions (front and side). This position causes the ch'i to scatter and become chaotic because of the different directions of traffic. Obviously, the impact is greater the more the roads are traveled. Deflective and absorbing remedies should be installed on both the front and side of the home with either a natural landscaping barrier such as hedges, or an artificial barrier such as a fence. Furthermore, install spotlights in the front yard and project the light source to the back of the home. This will help distribute the ch'i evenly and give the illusion the home is balanced on the lot.

A home positioned inside a U-bend gives the feeling and look of being encased in a noose. This lot position can create a feeling of being choked and may lead to feelings of anxiety. In addition, the inner bend of the curve will throw sha ch'i directly at the house when cars try to negotiate the curve. Just like a riverbed edge that corrodes with constant water movement, so too will the edges of the property erode that is constantly being bombarded with car sha. This is a difficult position to remedy, as the home is subjected to sha ch'i from the sides and front. High shrubbery like cypresses or arborvitaes planted in straight rows along the sides of the noose shaped road will protect and absorb the polluted ch'i. Placing reflective stones, lawn art, lighting, and objects of movement will also aid in deflecting the destructive energy.

A lot or home located at the tip of a sharp bend is referred to as a blade in feng shui road analysis. Cars will have difficulty negotiating the bend and may careen off the road into the property. Ch'i spins out of control resulting in haphazard ch'i entering the mouth of the home. As a result, the occupants may experience a great deal of chaos and confusion in their lives, making it difficult to focus and make decisions. Planting low thick hedging, or building a low brick wall, will act as a blockade to this destructive ch'i force. Adding fire elements (red colors, pointed shapes) in plantings and lawn art will represent the fire element, and as a result melt the metal blade (sickle) shape of the road design, thwarting the negative sha ch'i.

One of the best positions for a lot or home outside of a straight quiet road is the inside cradling position of an open U-junction. This road design has a gentle meandering curve where the lot sits on the inside of the curve and in essence is being cradled. This position protects the occupants from oncoming traffic, headlights, and poison arrows creating a benevolent ch'i to support the home and health of the occupants.

Obviously, there is a great deal that goes into choosing a property that will protect and ensconce the home with sheng ch'i. By and large, it is best to look for a location where the roadway has a gentle meandering curvature and not heavily traveled.

Other Environmental Factors Affecting Health

It is evident there are many different environmental factors that contribute to our well-being. In this section we will examine additional man-made structures that can have a negative impact on your health. Let's begin with assessing overly yin venues. Many times builders buy open plots of land that are in close proximity to a cemetery or ancient burial ground. These areas contain decaying ch'i, along with other facilities like mortuaries and funeral homes. It is inauspicious to purchase or build on a property that is located within the vicinity of these sites. The home is enfolded with this lackluster ch'i and as a result the occupants suffer from lethargy and potential ailments afflicting the weakest part of their body. Balancing this type of energy is very difficult since the energy vibration is substantially different from that of the living. It requires a trained dowser to identify the source, entrance point, and proper clearing techniques to adjust the vibration level. Although clearing techniques are helpful in abating this type of ch'i, it is not advisable to purchase in this type of location in the first place.

Garbage Dumps & Reclamation Centers

Garbage dumps and reclamation centers spew a disintegrating ch'i to the surrounding area along with pungent odors that can waft up to a one-mile radius. This type of ch'i lacks vitality and will have a negative impact on the residents over a period of time. It is advisable to research prior to purchasing a lot and maintain at least a two mile-radius from such a facility. If you realize your home is in close proximity to a garbage dump, then utilize good feng shui principles externally and internally including plantings of toxic absorbing plants such as philodendron, spider, golden pathos, brassica juncea, and yellow popular trees. Decorate your space on the yang side using lighter colors, movement objects, reflective materials, and bright lights. This will balance the overly yin ch'i that will otherwise surround your home.

Police Stations & Prisons

It is inadvisable to live near a police station, prison, or government facility that deals with crime issues. The ch'i associated with these sites is destructive and malevolent. The occupants living near these facilities will always be on guard for their personal safety. As a result, this can create a substantial amount of stress in their lives and predispose them to illness and disease. In order to gain a sense of security and allow the body to relax, plant a line of trees along side a fence and project a bright lighting source towards the roof of the house. This will give the illusion the house is grand and well protected.

Firehouses & Hospitals

Firehouses, hospitals, or psychiatric facilities also are considered inauspicious to live near. The loud sirens contribute to noise pollution, while the various ailments linked to hospitals saturate the surrounding ch'i with illness, injury, and unfortunate accidents. Blocking and deflective agents are recommended along with images of vitality and health placed within the immediate surrounding to balance the otherwise sickly ch'i.

Airports & Railways

Airports and railroads are extremely problematic to live near, especially if you are inside the traffic pattern. The constant noise pollution from overhead air traffic results in incessant arguing and restless sleep patterns. This combination contributes to a high stress load on the body and with time can compromise health. A railroad running directly behind the property will bathe the home with EMF's equivalent to a high-tension wire. This is an exorbitant amount of electromagnetism bombarding the home that can cause a host of ailments ranging from headaches, allergies, lethargy and hyperactivity in children. Both scenarios should be avoided since the cumulative effects can take its toll on the body. Those who find themselves in such a position will need to deflect and absorb the problematic ch'i. For overhead plane traffic, the only solution is to attach a reflective metal sheet to the attic ceiling to help bounce the sha ch'i from the home. Placing soothing sounds in your environment such as a waterfall fountain, aquarium, chime, or nature sounds can help to balance the otherwise harsh noise pollution. These remedies are minimal at best, and it is preferable not to purchase around these facilities. In the case of railroads, a natural barrier of pines or poplar trees will absorb some of the EMF emissions and block negative ch'i. Soothing sound remedies are also recommended to disguise the noise pollution. It is also advisable to avoid building or purchasing in areas surrounding these scenarios.

Factories & Businesses

Factories and businesses carry an overly yang ch'i energy and potentially toxic chemicals that can affect the surrounding air quality. These chemicals discharge positive ions into the air and as a result the percentage of bacteria and fungus increase. This is problematic and therefore an inauspicious site to build or purchase. To counteract the sha ch'i from this type of location, use natural barriers with landscape incorporating toxic absorbing plants (see pg. 87). Internally, incorporate natural elements along with salt lamps or salt candles. These items emit negative ions into the air and act as natural air purifiers.

Toxic Absorbing Plants

- <u>Philodendron, Spider & Golden Pathos:</u> absorb formaldehydes
- <u>Gerbera Daisies & Chrysanthemums:</u> removes benezenes
- <u>Dracaena, Massangeana, Spathiphyllum:</u> absorbs toxic vapors
- <u>Poplar Trees:</u> absorbs all toxins including pesticides
- <u>Rye, Fescue Grass:</u> absorbs toxins including pesticides
- <u>Sunflowers:</u> absorbs toxins including pesticides
- <u>Mulberry:</u> absorbs toxins including pesticides
- <u>Apple Trees:</u> absorbs toxins including pesticides

High Tension Wires & Cell towers

High-tension wires and cell towers are extremely problematic man-made structures that we encounter with modern day living. These structures emit EMF's and radiofrequency fields respectively. These frequencies vibrate at a much higher rate than the human alpha brain waves and therefore can potentially predispose individuals to an array of medical conditions ranging from general malaise, headaches, eye problems, dizziness, allergies, and ADD, to more serious diseases such as leukemia and other cancers. Since the fields dramatically decrease with distance, it is imperative a dwelling is at least 600 to 1000 feet from the source. It is extremely difficult to shield your home from these frequencies, but some protection can be achieved by planting poplar or pine trees around the property along with placing protective devices (see resource page) inside the home and directed at the offending wire or tower. Obviously, choosing a site without these structures altogether is best.

Parks & Schools

Living across the street from a park or school can disrupt the equilibrium of yin and yang. This occurs especially during peak and off-peak hours or time of year when activity will wax and wane disproportionately. Schools, in addition to having an overabundance of youthful ch'i that can lead to insomnia, anxiety, and muscle tension will also generate a disproportionate level of yin and yang energy depending on the particular time of day and school session. Furthermore, there is an elevated level of carbon monoxide fumes twice a day when buses transport students to and from the building. Therefore, when choosing a property, it is best to be located down the street from this type of ch'i, rather than directly across from it.

Places of Worship

Places of worship can be extremely peaceful and relate to spiritual growth; two attributes beneficial to life. However, there are also mixed energies that are associated with places of worship. Many times people resort to them during life challenges. The surrounding energy is imbued with these challenges. Occupants living in the vicinity are more likely to feel the pressures of this energy. When looking to purchase or build a home avoid locations in direct proximity to places of worship. If this is not an option, employ defective remedies.

Road Signs

Symbols have a way of impacting you on a conscious and subconscious level. When you are repeatedly exposed to them they become part of your psyche. If your home is positioned directly in front of a sign, then every time you enter and leave the dwelling you are patterned by the subliminal message of that symbol. Obviously, positive symbols or signs are beneficial, whereas those with negative connotations can create obstacles in your life. Below is a list of some common signs you may encounter and the impression they can make on your life.

1. <u>Dead End:</u> Looking at this sign on a daily basis reinforces the concept that your life is literally at an end and there is no place left to go. The subliminal message has a greater impact when you can visually see it from the home. In this case, the best solution is to conceal it through landscaping externally and drapery internally.

2. <u>Traffic Light:</u> If a traffic light is visible from the home the occupants may experience constant turmoil or have difficulty making decisions. The constant influx of people coming, going, or perhaps to stay, mimics the symbols of the lights (green) go, (red) stop, and (yellow), perhaps stay. This may be a bit more difficult to conceal, as the traffic light fixture can be quite high. Higher trees outdoors and adequate window treatment indoors will help to obstruct the view of the traffic light. Deflective and absorbing landscape measures should be installed to shield against car sha.

3. <u>Dip:</u> This sign in plain view to your home paints the pattern of life being filled with a roller coaster of ups and downs. The common reaction is a swing of emotions and that makes for very

stressful living. It's important to conceal the sign from plain view with landscaping and balance the polarities (yin/yang) on the interior and exterior of the home.

4. <u>Yield:</u> Programming the subconscious mind with this message tends to put the occupant in a subservient position to others. This is the individual who feels taken advantage of because they are literally yielding to others. In this scenario, it is important to make the environment more yang while concealing the sign.

5. <u>Arrows:</u> Any arrow directed to the house throws a piercing sha ch'i directly at the occupants. Depending on the area of the house that the constant affront is directed towards, it can manifest in the occupants lives as a personal challenge. Positioning a convex mirror to deflect the sha ch'i created by the arrow will counteract the otherwise spiraling ch'i.

The key behind signs and their subliminal messages is to shield them from plain view. In part, feng shui is a language of metaphors and symbols. Therefore, this is an important factor to take into consideration when analyzing a site for a dwelling.

Attacking Objects & Structures

Some objects and structures can present as a threat to the property based on the trajectory angle they form to the home. It is important to analyze the angles of neighboring roof lines, fences, cables, telephone poles, streets, edges of buildings, direction of pathways, driveways, street lamps, trees, etc. and determine if they are in direct alignment to the front door or rooms of vulnerability, such as the bedroom, kitchen, a gathering room, or home office. The penetrating force of ch'i created by the angles of these objects can be detrimental to the occupants. For example, a tree trunk, electrical pole, or street lamp that is in direct alignment to the front door or window presents as a direct attack to the mouth and eyes of the human body. In feng shui, the house is a replication of the human body, whereby the door represents the mouth and the windows represent the eyes. In addition to the bodily infraction, an object that obstructs these parts of the home will act as a barrier for the incoming ch'i and any opportunities that may come with it. This is why it is so important to plant trees with ample growing space, so when they mature, they don't become an obstacle or infringement to the home. When objects such as these are in direct alignment with the door or window, the best solution is to redirect the attacking ch'i upward and away from the mouth of the home. Placing a concave mirror above the doorframe or window tilted downward and in alignment with the tree, will redirect the powerful ch'i upward and away from the door or window. If the tree or pole is further away (60 plus feet), then a decorative trellis can be positioned in front to absorb and redirect the funneling ch'i.

Rooftops, Antennas, Buildings & Garage Doors

Rooftops, antennas, and sides of buildings can have a significant impact when homes are in clusters. Here you want to evaluate the relationship between the buildings. If one corner of a building or home is pointed directly towards the neighboring building, then the destructive funneling ch'i will show up as discord between the neighbors. In addition, potential health complaints may arise to the affected body part that corresponds to the part of the home with the affront. The best solution in this case is to plant soft hedging or to install a fence to absorb the funneling ch'i. You can soften the shape of the fence by planting climbers such as Clematis or Honeysuckle, as they have soft curving leaves. Planting Jasmine or Wisteria will provide a fresh scent for the surrounding area.

Larger buildings, driveways, and garages directly opposite the front door are also problematic. Anytime a larger building dwarfs a house, it is harmful to the occupants. The larger building absorbs the surrounding ch'i and therefore depletes it from the smaller home. It also emits a suppressive insurmountable energy, so the occupants of the smaller home feel overwhelmed. Planting columnar shaped trees or shrubbery, spotlights directed upward, and mounting a concave mirror to reflect a miniaturized image of the larger structure will in effect squash the overpowering feeling of the larger structure.

When a garage door or driveway is directly opposite of your front door the energy can be very threatening. The constant backing out of cars, and the awesome size of the garage doors opening and closing, sends a "killing ch'i" and "devouring ch'i" respectively. Planting higher hedges and landscaping is an excellent way to block the offending view and cushion the effects of this inauspicious alignment.

The Human Living Space

Disturbing Neighbors & Threatening Symbols

Disturbing neighbors are another factor to be aware of when analyzing a site. Whether it is physical debris, clutter, or general disarray of the yard, this disrupts the circulating ch'i within the area. Since you do not have control over another person's space, the best remedy is to block the offending site from your view by planting high hedging and other auspicious landscaping features. This will transpose the sha ch'i to sheng ch'i for entry into your personal space.

Finally, anything that has an obvious threatening symbol that is pointed directly at your house, translates into a direct attack. The easiest solution is to try and reposition the threatening object. If you are unable to do so, select beautiful landscape features and plant them in direct alignment to the offending agent to obscure the view.

All of these external factors directly impact the strength of the human body and its ability to thwart disease. The greater the threat derived from tainted soil, surrounding EMF's, sha road designs, problematic facilities, and land topography, the more resilient the negative vibrational energy pattern becomes. The negative energy pattern developed from these sources can directly contribute to individuals becoming ill and staying ill. This is part of the energy equation; unless it is altered to weaken and counteract the illness, recovery may be extremely slow or not at all.

The second part of this equation is the internal ch'i force of the home itself, as this directly influences the internal ch'i of the human body. In this next section, we will examine and evaluate all aspects of the house structure that can contribute to your overall health. In most cases, the home layout is constructed prior to moving in; therefore, a host of feng shui problems may exist that can impact health.

Human Body Perspective of The Home

Since the beginning of time man has searched for a protective site to call home. The ancient sages lived on the land using trees for protection first, then caves, and finally facades that were made from different locally available materials. These original basic houses took the appearance of the human face, with thatched roofs representing hair; openings for windows were positioned where the eyes and nose are on the face, and the door being a larger opening that would represent the mouth. The internal rooms represented the organs, whereas the walls that supported

The Feel-Good Home :: Feng Shui and Taoism for Healthy Living

and protected the rooms represented the skin. Feng shui looks at the structure of a house much in the same way as early man designed it. Every part of the home represents a part of the human body. This type of an analysis is based on the eight trigrams of the ba-gua, along with superimposing the human body vertically over the structure. By using the ba-gua we can assess many different types of health challenges.

If we examine the eight cells of the ba-gua, we can see that each gua has an associated body part. In general, the family sector oversees the feet, the wealth sector your hips, pelvis, and bones, the fame sector your eyes, the relationship area the internal organs, the children section the mouth area, the helpful people sector the head and lungs, the career sector the ears, the knowledge sector the hands, and the center oversees the overall health and other body parts. Below is the ba-gua depicting the basic guas and how to use it from three-door entry position, or as a directional compass. The Human Ba-gua Chart (page 93) provides additional areas of the body associated with each gua or sector.

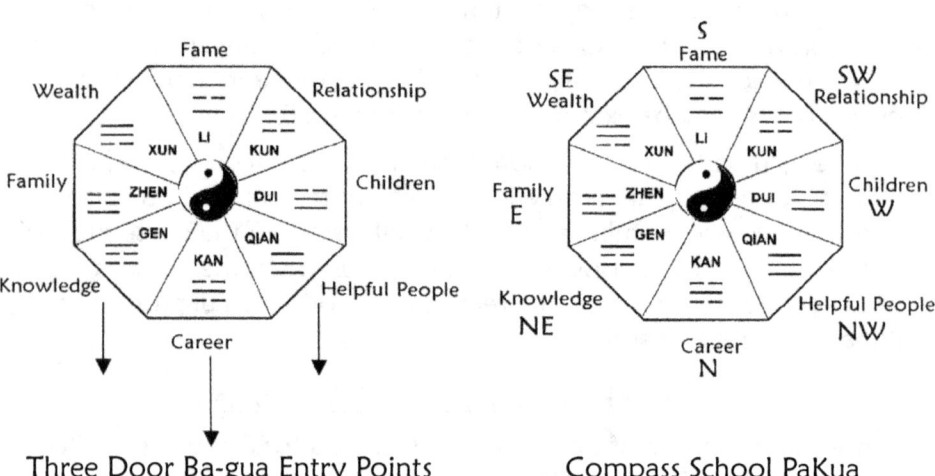

Three Door Ba-gua Entry Points
Fig. 23

Compass School PaKua
Fig. 24

The Human Ba-gua

- <u>Family:</u> (Zhen) Feet, liver, and gallbladder
- <u>Wealth:</u> (Xun) Thighs, hip, liver, gallbladder, waste, muscles, strong odors, and tendons
- <u>Fame:</u> (Li) Eyes, heart, tongue, small intestine, circulatory system, and sense of smell
- <u>Relationship:</u> (Kun) Abdomen, digestive system, spleen, stomach, and shoulders
- <u>Children:</u> (Dui) Mouth, teeth, lungs, large intestine, and skin
- <u>Helpful People:</u> (Qian) Head and lungs
- <u>Career:</u> (Kan) Ears, bladder, kidney, reproductive organs, spine, bone marrow, hair on head
- <u>Knowledge:</u> (Gen) Hands, fingers, stomach, and spleen

Architectural Shape

In feng shui the architectural shape has the greatest impact on health and overall success in life. Essentially, there are three basic guidelines that should be incorporated into the house shape. They are stability, balance, and smoothness. How stable and balanced a structure is depends upon its shape. A square or rectangular shape is considered the most auspicious design in feng shui. These shapes represent the earth and symbolize stability, dependability, and a sense of security. A square or rectangular shape that has more than one level should be balanced on each floor. In other words, one floor should not be larger or smaller than the other. The design should maintain a sense of smoothness, roundness or curvatures, as this aids in ch'i to flow smoothly while gracing the occupants with a nurturing feeling. Harsh angles or protruding corners should be avoided, as they cause the ch'i to move too harshly and can cause unexpected accidents or injury.

Irregular shaped architecture lacks stability and a sense of balance. If we understand that the human body and life experiences are encapsulated within the structure, then living in an irregular shape building results in depleted ch'i in body systems and the area of your life that corresponds to the missing gua(s). Unfortunately, most homes are designed with irregular shapes and therefore the owner takes on life challenges rooted into the structure. Feng shui applications can re-establish balance and revitalize depleted ch'i.

There are several options to choose from to rebalance an L-shape or meat cleaver shape home depending on the occupants' budget. Planning an addition to fill in the missing section will square the home off and bring it back into balance for ch'i to flow properly. This is obviously the most costly remedy. Installing a patio, deck, lamppost, bird feeder, or landscaping where the missing corner is, are all viable options in creating a sense of balance in the design and boosting the otherwise depleted ch'i. Internally, hang a mirror or scenic vista on the rear wall of the room that abuts the missing section to give the illusion of extending the room. Setting an intention with affirmations about gaining back the depleted ch'i in the corresponding body part and life aspect, and placing it behind the mirror or vista, can have a powerful affect in the overall cure.

Architectural shapes that are more challenging are the U-shape, S-shape, and triangular shape buildings. These designs are especially undesirable because they carry a great deal of destructive energy. In these scenarios, it is simply best to live elsewhere.

Homes designed with a steep roof pitch, or many small rooms protruding from the top of the house with dormer windows creates a harsh triangular structure and irregular roof. This is a destructive energy for the occupants, as the ch'i rises and escapes too quickly. In addition, the structure appears rather dominating, as if it were fighting with the sky or heavenly energy. Instead, roofs should take on a lower pitch or domed shape so the ch'i can modulate properly and remain in the structure for an appropriate time to feed and nourish the occupants.

Building Materials

Homes contain a vast amount of synthetic materials in their construction design. Waterproofing, foundations, carpets, flooring, adhesives, grouts, plastics, lighting, paints, wallpaper, furniture, fabrics, and insulation are just a few examples of potential irritants. These materials are irritating because of the volatile outgassing components released directly into the living space. Headaches, allergies, sinus ailments, and eye irritants are just some maladies that go hand-in-hand with synthetic outgassing. Let's face it; you can't totally avoid synthetics in your environment unless you choose to live in a bubble.

Your best recourse is to incorporate as many natural materials as you can into the design. Real hardwood, granite, slate, ceramic, stone, cotton and silk fabrics, organic paints, or those with low VOCs (Volatile Organic Compounds), bamboo, wicker, toxic absorbing plants, flowers, salt lamps, and proper ventilation are all examples of ways to counteract the negative effects of synthetic emissions. This is an extremely important factor to consider in home design to safeguard you and your family from potential illnesses.

Internal Structures

Doors, windows, and ceilings are other structural features that should be balanced. In feng shui, the doors correspond to the mouth area and represent the voice of the parents or authoritarian figure. The front door in particular represents who you are and is the primary point where ch'i energy enters. The size of the door should be proportionate to the overall structure, so ch'i does not seep out (overly large) or be stifled (overly small). The largest person in the home should fit comfortably through the door allowing the aura to expand freely. There should be a clear meandering path to the door wide enough to allow the ch'i and the human body to enter freely. The front entrance should be well lit, attractive in appearance, and fully functional. A door that is difficult to open, squeaky, or malfunctioning to any degree will result in miscommunication with the outside world, potential obstacles, and health challenges, especially to the urinary and kidney systems (north facing). Pay special attention to any attacking features, man-made or natural, and remedy them with blocking or deflective modalities.

The architectural design should allow for the front door to be in alignment with the rest of the structure and not recessed or difficult to find. A hidden door breeds uncertainty of your destination in life or a feeling to hide from the world. In such cases where the front door is hidden, it is important to give direction with a clear well-lit path, colorful landscape, and movement objects such as chimes, a fountain, or flag. The idea is to eliminate any ambiguity that otherwise is associated with a hidden door design.

The front door entrance should also be free of any heavy overhang or balcony above it. These designs leave the body feeling vulnerable to a possible collapse and injury. Large pillars across a front porch aligned in rows are also considered inauspicious, as it takes on a prison-like effect stifling your freedom. If they feel constricting when entering or exiting the front door, then simply place hanging plants to offset the confining design.

The door itself should open inward to allow full ch'i expansion. Solid wood is the preferred material, as it provides a sense of strength and protection while looking posh. Avoid front doors that are glass only, as they lack strength, durability, and privacy leaving the occupants feeling vulnerable and on display.

The foyer design should be open and airy to mimic the phoenix position to the front of the home. This provides a ming tang or open space for clear vision and expression in your life. When foyers are non-existent or small with an immediate wall in front of you, it translates as an obstacle causing the body to tighten up and the aura to contract. Keeping the area clutter free and placing a vase with flowers or a scenic vista will allow the body to relax and expand into the symbolic beauty.

The layout and positioning of internal doors can also have a direct impact on health. Doors that are misaligned across from each other, or disproportionate in size, create disturbances of the mouth region ranging from sensitive teeth, gingivitis (inflammation of gums), or jaw problems. This type of door positioning also contributes to poor communication, bickering, and potential divorces. The solution is to install a decorative lighting fixture, preferably one with reflective quality between the doors to offset the misalignment. If there are three or more doors in a small area, where one or more of these doors lead to the outside garage or basement, then vital ch'i can leak out of the home. Depending on where this configuration falls in the overall floor plan and ba-gua, it can weaken that body system (i.e.: north side of the structure, bladder and kidneys will be affected). The solution is to install a beautiful lighting fixture in the center where the doors converge to diffuse the ch'i.

When there are three or more doors positioned in a straight line, especially down the center of the home, ch'i will run too quickly and not be able to flourish and feed the center point. The center provides stability to the entire home and considered the heart of the structure. Disturbances here caused by fast moving ch'i can result in digestive and circulatory problems. This is exacerbated when the front door is also in alignment with these doors. The key is to redirect the ch'i and slow it down by placing objects in its path such as artwork, a carpet runner, crystal chandelier or plant.

Doors that are positioned too close in proximity and hit into each other when opened are referred to in feng shui as "arguing doors." As a result, the location where this occurs is also an area where the occupants tend to fight. Furthermore, the constant banging between the doors can result in toothaches and TMJ (temporomandibular joint-or jaw) disorders, since doors correspond to the mouth area. The best solution is to re-hang the doors so they do not open into each other. If this is not a viable solution, then be mindful of keeping the doors closed and open one door at a time when needed. There are other schools of feng shui that remedy this scenario through symbolism and intention. The suggestion is to symbolically bring the doors into harmony by tying a red string around both door-knobs and then cut the string to release any tension between the doors. Red only attracts positive energy; therefore, positive energy is now brought in as a truce between the doors and the family members respectively.

Finally, any doors that are blocked and cannot open or are physically missing can cause a host of problems ranging from missed opportunities, struggles, and overall challenges in life. The location of this door scenario in the overall ba-gua of the home will determine the potential ailment encountered by the occupant. It is best to de-clutter areas around any doorways and either hang new doors where they are missing, or remove hinge plates from moldings to eliminate the door entirely.

Double doors entering a home or into a room causes an overabundance of ch'i entering at one time. This can lead to anxiety, especially when this door design enters into a bedroom. The best solution is to keep one door locked at all times and, in the case of a front door, place a decorative wreath or plaque indicating which door to access.

Internal doors that are designed on an angle are highly problematic when opening into a bedroom. This is because the ch'i will inadvertently have a direct alignment to a portion of the bed and push energy too harshly against the aura during sleep. This can lead to anxiety and restless sleep. The best solution is to keep the doors closed at night and place a decorative piece of artwork on either side of the door to mitigate the angled feel of the room.

Those rooms in feng shui that are considered less important (laundry room, storage room, utility room) and are in direct alignment with important rooms (bedroom, family room, office) whose door jam is larger, tend to incite feelings of insignificance and lack of self-accomplishment. If this is the case, simply place a mirror on the side of the wall by the smaller door to give the illusion there is equality between the door sizes.

Finally, doors that open out towards you are highly problematic, as they pull ch'i out rather than allowing it in. This can cause respiratory ailments (literally taking the life breath away) and overall life challenges. Many times when doors are hung this way the entry point is to a sidewall. This causes the ch'i to be squeezed and can lead to shoulder, neck, and back problems. The best solution is to re-hinge the doors. If you are building or renovating your home, then do not have them designed this way.

In conclusion, all internal and external doors should function properly since they correspond to how you communicate on a personal and social level. Healthy doors translate into good communication, better relationships, and peaceful living.

Windows

Windows in feng shui correspond to the physical eyes and therefore provide a view to the outside world. They also represent the voice of the children. According to feng shui theory, there should be three windows to every door. If the ratio of windows to doors is skewed, with more windows, children will take control of their parents and struggles will ensue. It is not to say children should not be heard, as a matter of fact it is healthy for them to be able to develop their own identity separate from their parents.

We are looking to achieve a delicate balance between the child and parent where both will feel heard and respectful of one another. A simple remedy is to hang a large chime on an exterior door frequently used by the children. When they enter the home, the chime will sound and alert the parents while reminding the children of who is in charge.

When there is an overabundance of windows, or very large windows within a structure, the ch'i is more likely to escape depleting the overall energy within the space. The occupants will feel vulnerable and anxious because windows lack the strength, support, and security that walls otherwise provide. There is also a tendency that the occupants will feel they are on display for the entire world to see. This is especially true in today's building trends where floor to ceiling windows are the norm. This is a major feng shui faux pas since windows of that magnitude are out of balance. These huge window proportions also let in an enormous amount of sunlight making the room overly yang. As a result, this will draw on the occupants own yang energy making them feel overly tired. This situation is exacerbated if these windows are located on the western side of the home. Western light lacks ions and therefore creates a white light that can leave us feeling very drained. The best solution is to have adequate window coverage to shield the sunlight and provide coverage at night for privacy and a feeling of security.

It is essential to take an inventory of all the windows within the home, as they represent the physical eyes in the human body and how you literally view all things in the world. Any windows that are in disrepair, have torn or no screens, do not lock, are cracked, scratched, stuck or simply dirty need to be addressed, especially if any of the occupants are experiencing eye problems. Always begin your survey in the bedroom, as this room has the greatest impact on your health. Then proceed throughout the rest of the home assessing all windows. Should your space not have a window or door to the back of the home, this will cause the ch'i to stagnate and can cause dry eyes or dry mouth issues. The best solution is to create a faux window or door through a mural design. This will effectively give the impression of an opening to the back of the structure for energy to release.

Ceilings

The internal ceilings represent the head when the body is in a vertical standing position. They also represent points closest to the heavenly position in the home and have a tremendous impact on how ch'i flows throughout the space. By and large, ceilings that are flat or dome shaped are most auspicious since they allow the ch'i to flow and nourish the room properly. When ceilings are overly high (12-30 feet) nourishing ch'i will shoot upwards and become trapped at the top of the ceiling. This is problematic as there is a lesser concentration of ch'i source within the room. In order to give the illusion the ceiling is lower, place decorative molding or artwork horizontally across the room to trigger the eye to a more appropriate height (8-10 feet) where the body will feel more comfortable and the ch'i will redirect and circulate properly.

Overhead beams, although attractive in many designs, present a health issue especially when they are in bedrooms or rooms where a great deal of time is spent. When there is an outcropping of a design feature such as a beam, the right angle that is formed between the wall and the beam will cause a backflow of ch'i compressing it downward at a speed of 96 feet per second (gravity) and rain down on anything in its path. Should that be a bed beneath the beam, then whatever area of the body that is in direct alignment with that beam will absorb this pelting ch'i and over time the result is discomfort or potential injury to that area of the body. The easiest solution is to reposition the bed, desk, or chair from beneath the beam. If this is not an option, the traditional remedy is to place two bamboo flutes with red tassels on the beams in a diagonal with the mouthpieces facing down. The bamboo represents flexibility and strength, while the angled object works to shift the ch'i upward. Using decorative brackets, painting the beams the same color as the ceiling, or placing inset lighting, are all viable options in redirecting the ch'i to a more beneficial movement.

Inverted "V" ceilings that slope downward are also problematic designs since they constrict ch'i flow causing a suppressing feeling. These are problematic when sleeping or working under as the constriction of ch'i and pressure can cause headaches and neck aches. The best solution is to reposition the bed or work area. The second option is to elevate the ch'i with upward lighting, terminating crystals points (pointed quartz crystals), or upward artwork.

Ceilings in main rooms that have skylights or that vary in heights can also present difficulties. A skylight is like being viewed and examined under a microscope. This can be unnerving over a bed or desk. If positioned over a desk, the added sunlight can be overwhelming as it beats down on top of the head. Skylights are more appropriate in rooms that are darker in color or in social rooms because they will furnish more light and create yang energy, which is appropriate for such a room scenario. If a skylight is already a part of the home design, hanging a faceted crystal from it will reflect the light and spread a rainbow of colors throughout the room. Do not hang the crystal if the skylight is in the bedroom, as the crystal is too energetic and will interfere with sound sleep. Instead, it is best to install a window treatment system that can cover the sky window at night and shield the moonlight. This is an important factor as it is essential there is total darkness in the bedroom for a reparative sleep state to ensue.

Ceilings that vary in heights from room to room will cause the human aura to expand and contract continually. It is uncomfortable for the body to be under this type of a constant change. Position higher furniture, upward lighting, terminating crystals, or artwork with upward movement on the side with a lower ceiling. Lower furniture, downward spot lighting, and artwork with a downward movement should be placed on the side with the higher ceiling. The eyes will interpret the uneven ceiling heights as balanced so the auric body can relax.

Finally, ceilings that are lower than eight feet in height will feel suppressive and constricting to the body. The feeling of being boxed in will lead to anxiety and general discomfort. Use bright lighting that is upward in design, lower pieces of furniture, and tall plants to drive the energy upward and give the illusion of height in the room. As a result, this will make the room feel more comfortable.

Hallways & Stairs

Hallways and stairs are the purveyors of ch'i within a house or building. They connect one room to another and one floor to another taking us to our destination point. Depending on the design and placement of the hallway or staircase will determine if the ch'i is auspicious or destructive. It is best if there are not too many hallways or stairs within the home, as the ch'i will become unmanageable. Homes that have long narrow hallways aligned from the front door to the back door, or directly aligned to bedroom doors, can be quite problematic. In these scenarios, the ch'i races from one point to another so quickly that it is unable to nourish any other points surrounding it. In this case, it is important to slow the energy by placing objects in its path such as hallway runners, artwork or a mirror on the wall, sconce lighting, plants, or a crystal chandelier. If the hallways are winding around the home, it will cause a twisting motion in the ch'i and can predispose the occupants to dizziness. Since all hallways are conduits of ch'i energy, it is important they are well lit and remain clutter free. Any clutter in a hallway will shut down ch'i movement into other areas of the home, much like a blocked meridian in the human body shutting down vital ch'i flow and nourishing oxygen to the organ site. It also will represent obstacles we might incur while traveling in the outside world.

Stairs are also conduits of ch'i connecting one floor to another. Therefore, just like hallways, staircases must be well lit and clutter free in order to be effective in distributing nourishing ch'i. When evaluating staircases the design and location is extremely important. The positioning of them is a distinguishing point between healthy ch'i and destructive ch'i. A spiral staircase may look architecturally appealing; however, in feng shui terms, it causes the ch'i to funnel creating a corkscrew effect that pierces the home. In addition, spiral staircases with open footings lack stability. As a result, humans as well as animals are hesitant to ascend and descend them. It is best not to incorporate a spiral staircase in a home design, but if it is pre-existing, then you can provide a sense of stability by placing a soft rounded plant and a spotlight beneath the stairs. Furthermore, positioning a bright light at the top of the staircase shining down will also aid in softening the problematic effects.

Staircases located in the center of the home pierce the heart, destabilizing the structure. Occupants can experience cardiovascular or respiratory illness as a result. In such a design scenario, anchor the staircase with earth elements or artwork with mountain scenes. Earth is considered a grounding element that can effectively anchor this otherwise destabilizing energy.

Stairs that are aligned to the front door or to a bedroom are also problematic in feng shui. First, ch'i is sucked up to the second floor before it has a chance to meander and nourish the first level. This action creates confusion in the direction of ch'i flow causing ch'i from the second floor to rush down and straight out the front door compromising the finances and general well-being of the occupants. If a bedroom is at the top of a staircase ch'i will rush into the room creating pressure. The best solution is to capture and redirect the ch'i from the door entry position. Depending on the foyer entry size, remedies can range from a circular patterned rug with a table and floral arrangement, to a crystal chandelier, plants, an interesting throw draped over the banister, a carpet runner with brass inset rails, a wall mural design, or artwork along the staircase wall. Finally, always keep the bedroom door closed at night to block and deflect the incoming ch'i.

Narrow steep staircases will cause ch'i to move much too quickly causing an overwhelming rush of energy. Stairs that are steep will also appear daunting to climb and descend. In order to counteract the steep vertical pitch, hang artwork to create a horizontal line on the wall that the stairs run. This will balance the vertical pitch and slow down the ch'i by providing objects for it to bounce off of.

Another staircase design that is problematic is the split staircase. Here the stairs go up on one side and down another. The ch'i is split in either direction disrupting its natural movement. In essence, the body also becomes confused as to which direction to move in. The solution is to direct the ch'i flow in one distinct pattern. Incorporating decorative artwork or a lighting fixture with reflective qualities in the landing area can achieve this. Furthermore, the aforementioned cures will provide a focal point for the human body and aid in ch'i flow.

Open Floor Plan & Structural Corners

Home designs with expansive open floor plans lack internal walls. This is problematic, as walls create boundaries from one room to another and without a sufficient amount of walls the body feels exposed and unsupported. In addition, the ch'i has free reign and as a result will move chaotically throughout the space. This in turn contributes to chaos and unclear thinking for the occupants. To contain the energy, create faux walls by utilizing plants, decorative screens, or boxes. This will give the impression of a barrier between rooms and restore the ch'i to a normal meandering flow.

Pillars and structural corners can cause an affront to a portion of the room they are located in. Depending on the position of the angled structure in the room and its corresponding gua, blocked energy can occur in that life sector and body part for the occupants (see the Human Ba-gua chart). If the pillar is square, like a structural corner, the 90-degree angle will cause the ch'i to project in a spiraling motion and bombard anything within its path. If it is a place where the occupant spends a great deal of time, the result is pain in the area of the body that is in direct alignment to this angled architecture. To soften the ch'i flow, simply place either a draping fabric, flowing plant, or any object between the angled projection and the occupant. The object will absorb the spiraling ch'i as opposed to it being absorbed by the human body.

Fireplaces

Fireplaces are wonderful architectural accents that imbue a room with ambiance and warmth. In feng shui, fire is the most powerful element. Because of this, it can have a negative impact for the occupants. When it is positioned in the center of a room or the center of the overall structure, beneficial ch'i will be sucked up the flue, while the fire itself can cause the occupants to feel "burnt out." If the location is in the center of the home, the best balancing modality is to place earthy objects (terra cotta, stone, ceramic, tan or brown colors) around it. In the five elemental concepts, the earth will drain the fire element and reduce the effects of the fire energy.

When fireplaces are located elsewhere, water features (water scene, mirror, glass vase) can be placed near the fireplace to keep the fire element under control. Avoid using the water feature if it is in the center of the home or located in the south direction of the home since it is in conflict with these points.

Positioning of Rooms

The layout of rooms within the overall floor plan is a key element behind a healthy flowing ch'i pattern. This translates into good health and prosperous living. Essentially, the front side of the house in feng shui is considered to be the yang side or social sector of the home. Rooms that are considered yang or social are the living room, dining room, or an office. When we think about socializing with people or doing business, we are reluctant to bring them to the back of the home or second floor, as these areas are more personal and take on a yin position in the home. From another perspective, the first room that you see upon entering the home triggers the body into a thought process about the purpose of the room at that moment and will program your desires. For example, if the first room is a kitchen, then thoughts are about eating. If it is a bedroom, it's about resting. A bathroom, well that speaks for itself, and an office will program the mind to work. It is best for a living room to be the initial presentation since it exudes an uplifting social feeling. That is certainly a wonderful energy to walk into on a daily basis.

Kitchen

The location of a kitchen is extremely important in feng shui, as this room represents your health and your overall ability to feed your family. This room should be well protected and not visible from the front entrance. When entering the kitchen, it is important there is full view of the room and not a partial or split view. The doorway should not be too narrow otherwise the ch'i will funnel and create a negative energy. There should also be more than one door entrance into this room to ensure good ch'i circulation. This room should be centrally located in the home for easy access, but not positioned through the center point of the home.

The center of the ba-gua relates to overall health and stability. The fire element of the kitchen will excite the earth element that is associated with the center point and cause agitation to organ systems such as the stomach and intestines, two organs that correspond to the center point of the home. The cooking area should be symmetrical and offer a full view of the door entrances so a command position can be achieved. This will allow the body to remain calm and relaxed. Avoid any overhead racks in the cooking area, as fear of collapse and injury can leave the body tense. Finally, a bathroom should not be positioned in the kitchen or abut it. These two rooms are diametrically opposed in purpose and inauspicious to commingle. Furthermore, the elemental components of these two rooms are constantly at war (kitchen-fire, bathroom-water). This may predispose the occupants to digestive problems and discord during meals.

Bathrooms

Bathrooms are one of the most challenging room placements in feng shui. Historically, this room was never placed within the dwelling, as the energies associated with it were considered inauspicious. By and large, this was due to archaic plumbing techniques. Today, our plumbing capabilities allow for proper waste lines, not to mention that fixtures can be quite dramatic and even luxurious. Even so, the bathroom in feng shui is still regarded as a draining energy source to the home and therefore placement in any gua is problematic, with certain areas having a more detrimental effect on your health and livelihood. Bathrooms that are located in the center of the home or the center of a room have the most killing ch'i effect on your health. The unstable energy associated with this room will in turn destabilize and exhaust the earth element that is associated with the center point and can affect your health and finances. The finances can become unstable because in feng shui water is associated with money and water within the bathroom is constantly draining out through the flushing of toilets, or water down the sink, shower or tub drains. Bathrooms will have a draining effect on any life station (gua) within the home with the greatest impact on areas such as relationships, health, wealth, career, and reputation. Feng shui remedies are necessary to counteract this otherwise draining energy source (see chapter 7). Finally, bathrooms should not be positioned over an entranceway, in direct line of the front door, or abut to a bedroom wall that the head of the bed is placed on. They also should not be in a kitchen, above a kitchen or eating area, or at the end of a long hallway. (See chapter 7 for further details).

Bedrooms

The bedroom is considered another room in feng shui that has the greatest impact on your health and overall livelihood. People spend anywhere from six to ten hours a day in this room sleeping. This is a passive or yin activity and therefore these rooms are best positioned in the yin side of the home (back or upper level). There should only be one entrance into the bedroom otherwise circulating nourishing ch'i will escape. The door should not face a stairwell, especially one that leads to the entrance point of the home. The energy is too powerful and will have a negative impact on the individual. There shouldn't be any exposed beams, a slanted ceiling, or irregular shape to the room. It is best if there is not a bathroom attached to this room or a bathroom positioned directly above it. The bedroom should not be along side or above the kitchen, at the end of a long hallway, in a basement, above a garage, or beneath the front entrance. These locations can have a negative impact on the body during sleep. (Refer to chapter 7 for further details).

Garage

The garage placement is important in relation to the key rooms (bedroom, kitchen, home office) within the home and can have a tremendous impact on your health and safety. Theoretically, the best position for a garage is detached from the living quarters since the space is generally utilized for storage of chemicals (paints, gasoline, oil, etc.) or sharp tools. These objects can have a negative impact on your health if you sleep or work above or along side them. When the garage is attached to the home it becomes part of the overall floor plan. Therefore, when superimposing the ba-gua over the structure a specific part of your life and body system will reside in this area. The potential toxins, sharp tools, broken items, or clutter so commonly associated with this space become the level of ch'i associated to that part of your life or organ system. If the garage is attached to the rest of the dwelling, the best location would be to the side of the house that doesn't have a living space adjoining it. If this is not a viable solution, then have the garage abut a room that is used infrequently such as a laundry room, storage closet, or utility room.

These rooms will act as a good buffer to the more functional living spaces. Finally, it is best a garage is not designed to be the focal point or front feature of the home, especially if the doors are more prominent looking than the front entrance. In this scenario, the occupants will be literally driven in life and become a slave to the car rather than the car serving them. If this is the case, then draw the attention to the front entrance with beautiful landscaping, decorative pots, wreaths, or chimes to detract from the garage doors.

Property & Driveway

The first part of this chapter was all about the land and what to look for. The front, backyard, and driveway now become part of the overall feature and design. They literally act as buffers to the outside and inside ch'i. First, the backyard should be a bit larger than the front, meaning the house is positioned just about in the middle of the property, hedging closer to the front yard. The property should always be well maintained, have variations of vegetation in species, height, and color. A lovely water feature in the front will collect ch'i and provide a beautiful view or ming tang. Curving pathways to the front entrance will allow the ch'i to gently meander into the home. The home should be positioned so the driveway across the street is not directly aligned to the front entrance. There should not be a pole, large tree, overly large structure, problematic road design, or any other attacking features directed at the home. It is wise to have buffering features to the front of the home such as a trellis, garden, landscaping, or even a porch to protect against any of the aforementioned negative factors. Other items that may be incorporated as accent features such as bridges, landings, verandas, decks, gazebos, or pools should be assessed for their size and placement in relation to the home. For example, decorative landscape bridges should entice ch'i flow from one pathway to another. The ch'i should flow smoothly to allow the human body to settle and relax. Furthermore, the bridge's position should be offset in relation to the rear door entrance. This type of an alignment will prevent ch'i from funneling directly into the home. Any type of decking, balconies, or verandas on second levels should be well supported with plantings and lighting beneath to act as a cushion. Gazebos or other decorative structures should retain a curving or circular design so ch'i can modulate smoothly around them.

Finally, pools should be size appropriate to the yard, curved in design, and positioned far enough away from the dwelling. If it is too close, the yin component of the contained body of water will pull the natural yang energy from the dwelling and, as a result, the occupants may feel drained. If the pool is positioned close to the back of the home, it will need to be balanced by the opposite polarity, or yang objects. Placing upward spotlighting, bright flowers, a gazing ball, reflective stones and objects will elevate the ch'i and balance the overly yin component of the pool.

Superimposing The Human Body Vertically To The Structure

In addition to superimposing the ba-gua over the structure or the individual room to assess the corresponding body systems, the human body can be positioned vertically within the entire structure or an individual room. By doing this we can assess the levels of the home and correspond them to the human body. For example, the lower level or basement of the home corresponds to the lower region or trunk of the body that contains the urinary system, colon, bladder, kidneys, large intestines and legs. The middle level corresponds to the main level of the home and relates to the middle region or torso that contains the spleen, stomach, gallbladder, pancreas and small intestine. The upper floors of the home correspond to the upper region of the body that contains the chest, heart, circulatory system, neck, and head. When there is a body system that is compromised, it is important to find the associated location within the home either by way of vertical superimposition of the body, or by the ba-gua method. Begin your assessment by checking the overall shape of the room, entire home and yard. If it is odd shaped, see if the missing section corresponds to the weakened body system. Check for any clutter, broken objects, nonfunctioning windows or doors, broken window panes or screens, peeling paint, holes in the walls, floor boards ajar, light bulbs that are blown or missing, dead space, dead vegetation, or garbage. Repair or refurbish anything you notice to be amiss. While doing this, set an intention that you are healing the section of your body that is associated with the areas you are cleaning or repairing.

The center of each room should also be evaluated since it is the point of all body systems and general health. Make sure to remove any clutter that might be in the center of a room. Less is more when it comes to the center point of a room. Repair any broken light fixtures; peeling paint on the ceiling, water stains from a prior leak, missing light bulbs or ones that are burnt out. Replace old furniture, worn rugs or flooring. Once you have made these adjustments, cleanse the space with essential oils and place a healthy plant to symbolize healing of the body system.

The ch'i of your body is interconnected with the ch'i of the dwelling. It is influenced on a daily basis by your immediate surroundings. Therefore, learning how to detect good ch'i flow in and around your dwelling can help to uncover potential blockages, stagnation, or destructive energy that over time can break down body systems. Sending positive vibrational energy yourself will attract those energies back to you and open your mind, body, and spirit to a healthy and balanced environment.

*The concepts discussed in this chapter can be found in many feng shui resources and training programs, as it is common practice when assessing and rectifying potential sha ch'i and architectural designs.

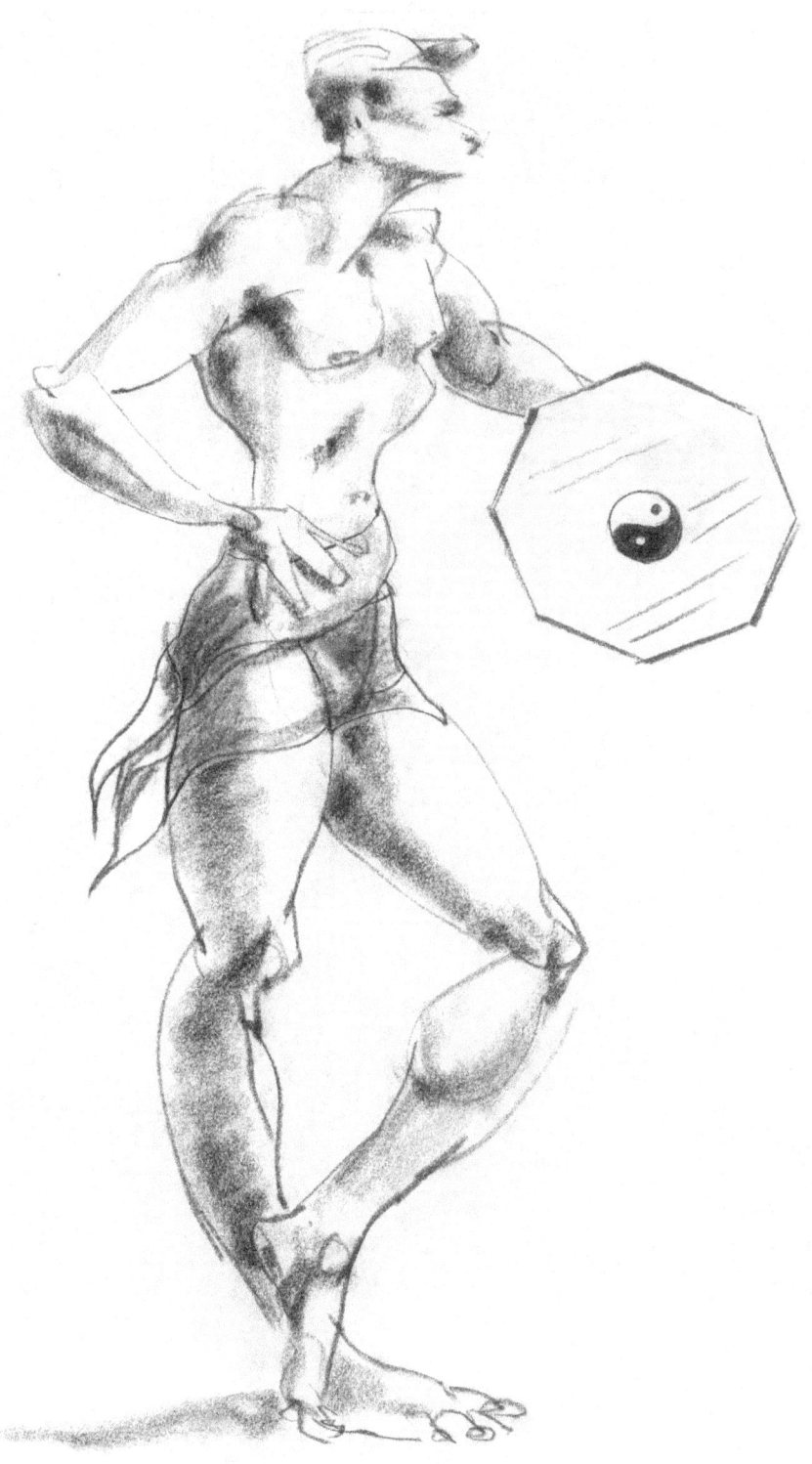

6

The Symbolic Ba-gua

"By nature, men are nearly alike; by practice, they get to be wide apart."

Confucius

The legendary emperor King Fu Xi (Hsi) discovered the ancient symbols known as trigrams in 3300BC. These trigram symbols represent great knowledge and wisdom regarding phenomena that affects life and the nature of the universe. They are mankind's legacy handed down by the ancient sages, as well as the building blocks of all Chinese philosophy, the I Ching, Astrology, Mathematics, Chinese Traditional Medicine, Numerology, Martial Arts and Feng Shui.

These markings that were rearranged by Yu the Great created a symmetrical shape with nine separate segments. Each segment contained a specific number ranging from one to nine. The even numbers are considered yin, and are placed to the corners of the square. The odd numbers are considered yang, and are placed at the four cardinal points and the center. The numbers nine and one are considered the most auspicious since nine represents wholeness or completion and one represents the beginning of all things. The central square representing the number five is the most powerful, as it is translates as "wu" for "mid-day" and "myself." The four quarters represent the four seasons and cardinal directions, while the four corners represent the inter-cardinal points. When adding the numbers horizontally, vertically, or diagonally they add to the number fifteen. This configuration was considered so auspicious that many countries such as China, Egypt, India, and Ireland built their cities with this configuration. The four quarters would represent the four quarters to a city and the middle square corresponded to the government building.

Wood	Fire	Earth
4	9	2
Southeast	South	Southwest
Wood	Earth	Metal
3	5	7
East		West
Earth	Water	Metal
8	1	6
Northeast	North	Northwest

Magic Square
Fig. 25

The numbers following in a clockwise position mimic the seasons and ratio of yang to yin. During the winter, yang is at its lowest (1) and yin is at its highest (8). During the summer, yang is at its highest (9) and yin is at its lowest (2). Imperial palaces were built specifically with these nine areas in order to depict the energy movement of the seasons. As a result, the emperor would spend a short period of time in each room of the palace according to its highest energy point. He did this so his rule was auspicious over his subjects. Each of the nine cells also represented the five elemental qualities believed to be the components of everything on earth, including man. The dynamic interplay between yin and yang gives rise to the eight trigrams, or eight great forces of nature.

The process begins with the great ultimate or Taiji giving birth to one yang bit and one yin bit. The yang bit represents change and the yin bit represents matter.

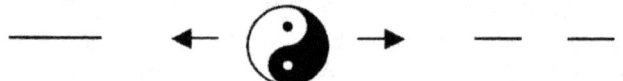

Individually, yang and yin each produce two offspring known as bigrams that represent an interrelationship between heaven and earth.

The bottom lines correspond to the parent polarity (yang or yin) and represent the earth position. The top line is a result of the production of the four unique bigrams (alternating yang and yin) and represents the heaven position. Each of the four bigrams gives rise to two trigrams each.

The Symbolic Ba-gua

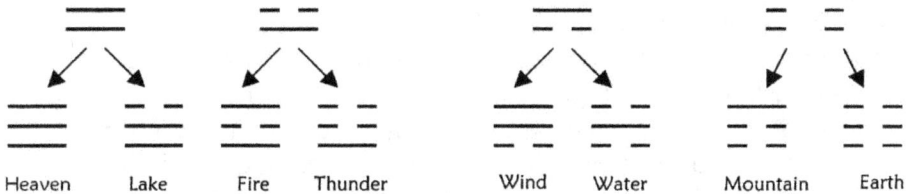

| Heaven | Lake | Fire | Thunder | Wind | Water | Mountain | Earth |

The third line added in the middle of each combination represents humanity. Hence, the three lines become the trinity of heaven (top), man (middle), and earth (bottom). These three line configurations, built from the bottom up, represent the eight natural forces of the universe. Each of these forces has their own ch'i vibration, color, element, family member, personality, related illness, and number.

In chapter three, it was noted that according to your birth data you have a greater affinity to one of the nine palaces or trigrams. Primarily, you keep these qualities throughout life, but over time you experience the other palace qualities. This occurs because the solar system is in a constant state of movement. This flux of energy can be traced on the magic square and can indicate the type of ch'i present over time. The benefit on a personal level is that you are able to experience the qualities of all the trigrams. This enables you to be exposed to various opportunities or potential obstacles.

Each trigram has a unique ch'i vibration and can impact your own ch'i according to the calculated kua number (Birth Trigram Calculation-Chapt. 3). Below is a list of the ch'i vibrational qualities of the trigrams.

Ch'i Vibration of Trigrams

- <u>Zhen (3) Thunder:</u> Movement, arousing, impulsive
- <u>Xun (4) Wind:</u> Gentleness, penetrating, flexible
- <u>Li (9) Fire:</u> Independent, adherence, clinging, precise
- <u>Kun (2) Earth:</u> Receptive, yielding, trusting, open
- <u>Dui (7) Lake:</u> Joy, satisfied, serenity
- <u>Qian (6) Heaven:</u> Initiator, strong, creative
- <u>Kan (1) Water:</u> Unreliable, cautious, dangerous
- <u>Gen (8) Mountain:</u> Patient, quiet, still, steady

The eight trigrams are configured differently depending on the interpretative ba-gua (Earlier Days format and Later Days format). The first interpretation (Earlier Days-see fig.2, chapt.1) is based on a time period when the earth was being formed. It represents the newborn baby's entrance into this plane bringing with it a childlike essence of wonder and innocence. It is a perfect model of harmony as seen by the positions of the trigrams in exact opposite polarities. In this configuration, Qian is found at the top because it represents heaven and the metal element. Metal is a result of the stars becoming a super nova and, since the stars are positioned in the heavens, this is an accurate trigram position. Kun is positioned beneath Qian and receives the penetrating forces of the heavens including the radiations from the sun and planetary bodies. Li is positioned to the east representing the fire energy of the sun. The sun rises in the east and sets to the west acting as a major point of reference for the ancient sages when configuring time, seasons (vernal equinox), and compass points. Therefore, this is a logical position for the Li trigram. The trigram Kan sits to the west directly across from Li. This is a logical position since the moon, represented by the Kan trigram, rises in the west where the sun sets. The earth reacts to the moon's magnetism by the rise and fall of the ocean tides; hence, the water energy of this trigram. Zhen and Xun sit diagonally across from each other on the intercardinal points. They represent wood energy and the natural forces of thunder and wind. A combination of these qualities fuels life through photosynthesis and the rain that is formed from the wind and thunder forces. Gen and Dui are the final two forces diagonally across from each other. The mountain energy of Gen is a result of movement beneath the earth's crust. The valleys along side the mountains collect rain and form the waterways (lakes, oceans, ponds) on this planet.

The Later Days ba-gua arrangement (see fig.4, chapt.1) represents a time when heaven and earth are clearly distinguishable. There is movement of the trigrams following the sequence of events in a lifelike world depicting the seasons, compass directions based on the apparent movement of the sun across the sky, time of day, and the human journey through life. This ba-gua arrangement is primarily used in feng shui practice and theoretically used indoors only. The Earlier Days system is still used today and should be applied to outdoor spaces. This does require a trained practitioner to compare the two systems during an analysis. However, many apply the Later Days ba-gua with great success.

The Symbolic Ba-gua

The Ba-gua Map

In feng shui, the ba-gua is primarily used to identify the areas of our life and the impact that changing ch'i forces have on us. The best way to ascertain just how your space is impacting you is to analyze it from the ba-gua perspective. The life map (ba-gua) can be superimposed over the entire structure, individual room, or both. In Compass School feng shui, the map is superimposed over the building using compass points and is referred to as the Pakua. In other schools of feng shui (Black Hat Sect and Western), the map is superimposed via door entry position and referred to as the ba-gua. If you use the map from door entry position and compass points, a room and or a building can potentially have two locations for each life area or gua. For example, there can be two separate areas for the relationship gua within a room or the entire structure. In some situations these two points will end up in the same position (ie: the far right corner of a room might also be the Southwest direction). When this occurs, then that area is extremely powerful in its effects.

When aligning the ba-gua map, it is best to superimpose it over an architectural floor plan or one that is drawn to scale. When utilizing it via three-door entry, simply superimpose it over the main door entrance of the home (either far right, middle, or far left-indicated by arrows).

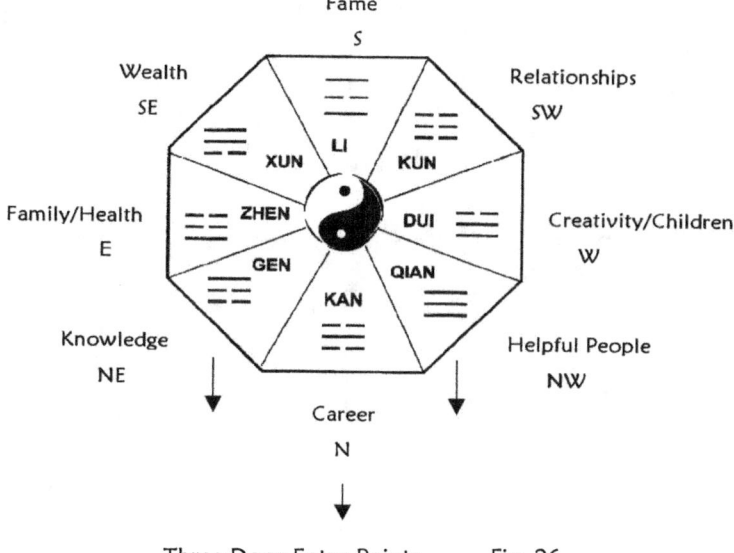

Three Door Entry Points   Fig. 26

When superimposing the map via compass direction follow the steps below:

1. Determine the facing direction of the home by utilizing a compass and standing with your back to the front door while looking out towards the street. Most of the time the front door is the facing direction; however, if it is hidden, or takes a more tortoise position, then look for the wide-open space for your facing point.
2. Take an architectural floor plan of your home or one drawn to scale.
3. Mark the 8 compass points on the floor plan (create 8 pie-wedges).
4. Superimpose Pakua over floor plans aligned with directions.
5. Note those areas of the home that correspond to the life aspirations.

In either method, make sure the entire structure encompasses the ba-gua map. This includes the garage only if it is attached to the overall structure. You may find that parts of the map will fall outside the structure if the shape of the building is irregular (see below).

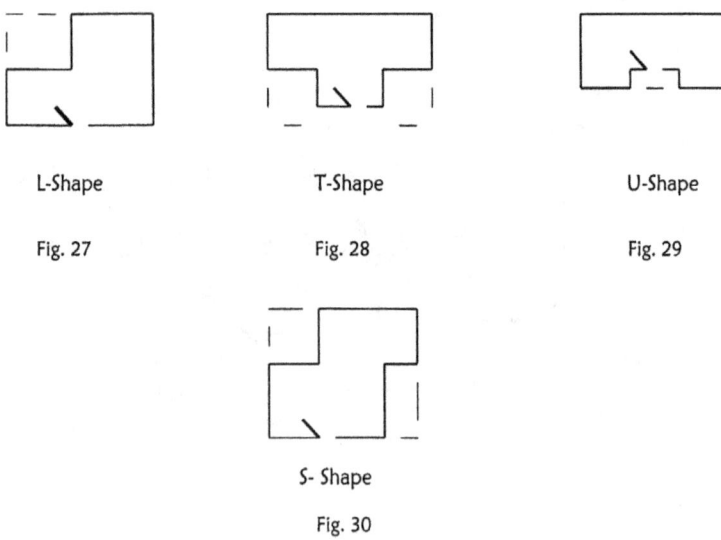

L-Shape   T-Shape   U-Shape

Fig. 27   Fig. 28   Fig. 29

S- Shape

Fig. 30

The Symbolic Ba-gua

When superimposing the ba-gua over an individual room, either align it to the door entrance to the room, or via compass direction. If there is more than one door entrance, you must choose the one that is used most frequently. Once again, make sure the entire room is encapsulated within the ba-gua. If the room has an odd shape, part of the ba-gua will fall outside of the room, just as it did with the overall structure. If you determine in either case that there are areas of the ba-gua that are missing due to the architectural shape, then filling in those areas symbolically will effectively boost the otherwise depleted ch'i. As mentioned in chapter five, the following solutions are effective in squaring off an irregular design.

<u>Internal:</u>

- Mirrors
- Terminating crystal points
- Scenic vista
- Symbolic artwork for the missing gua

<u>External:</u>

- Fence
- Deck
- Patio
- Landscaping
- Lamp post
- Bird feeder
- Sculpture
- Water feature
- Flag pole

<u>Mapping Out The Symbolic Ba-gua</u>

In this section we will examine how symbolic images can uplift the ch'i within a space and ultimately improve your well-being and life experiences. Through symbolic association you can program the mind and body positively. This is why it is so important that the objects you choose for your space are things you love and make sense to you. Dr. Wayne Dyer explains this concept in his third principle for getting everything you want in his book "Manifest Your Destiny." This principle states that you are an environorganism. What he means by this is you are an extension of your environment and cannot separate yourself from it. Once you realize you are part of the whole, it commands respect for everything you encounter. When you can respect what appears external to you, you begin to build a relationship of harmony, rather than trying to control what is outside of you.

One of the most important aspects to this principle is creating a space that is sacred. Filling your home with beautiful objects, the life forces of nature in plants, flowers, and animals are all components that contribute to designing a sacred space. Spending time in your environment and seeing it as a holy place, will allow you to feel spiritually connected, whole, and content. Knowing this puts you in touch with the laws of attraction bringing more positive energy into your life. Let us begin then to examine the life stations of the ba-gua and what images, symbols, and colors resonate to them.

<u>Zhen (3) Family/Health:</u> This gua is located at the middle one-third of the left wall via door entry or between (67.5-112.5) compass points. This gua has all the energy of the rising sun, the spring season, and the intensity of thunder energy. It represents the family heritage and strong physical health. These two dynamics provide a stable foundation to enjoy life and prosperity. This gua helps you to understand your roots, dreams, and aspirations for your family. It is the energy of the tree trunk from where your personal growth begins. This section can be enhanced with the following:

- Green and blue colors
- Wood elements
- Family heirlooms
- Family photo
- Symbols of famous people you respect
- Healthy plants and flowers
- Cultural heritage pieces
- Books on health and nutrition
- Artwork depicting health and vitality (field of poppies, vineyard, etc.)
- Exercise equipment (room appropriate)
- Columnar shapes and patterns
- Place herbs and essential oils for health
- Place animals of longevity such as a tortoise or crane
- Affirmations regarding a strong healthy body, mind, and soul along with healthy family relationships

<u>Enhancing Elements:</u> Wood and Water
<u>Detrimental Elements:</u> Fire, Earth, Metal

The Symbolic Ba-gua

<u>Xun (4) Wealth & Prosperity:</u> This gua is located to the far left hand corner via door entry or between (112.5-157.5) compass points. The penetrating, yet gentle energy that exudes from this gua, is all about the slow and steady pace to shape your wealth and resources in life. This may come in the form of good friends, good health, wealth, or an overall enjoyable life. It is about aligning yourself with your soul's purpose and, as a result, abundance will follow. This section can be enhanced with the following:

- Blue or green color hues with touches of purple or red
- Thriving plants especially a jade plant as it represents growth of finances
- Movement objects (chimes, flag – outdoors only), bird or sailboat images to generate wind ch'i
- Valuable artwork or possessions
- Water features like fountains will keep abundance flowing
- Aquarium or pictures of water flowing
- Objects of desire
- Coin collection
- Wood elements and columnar shapes or patterns
- Hang a faceted crystal to generate energy to this gua
- Affirmations confirming abundance on all levels in your life

<u>Enhancing Elements:</u> Wood and Water
<u>Detrimental Elements:</u> Fire, Earth, Metal

<u>Li (9) Fame & Reputation:</u> This gua is located in the middle one-third of the back wall upon door entry or between (157.5-202.5) compass points. It represents the fire image, independence, precise nature, and clinging ch'i. This gua depicts your reputation in the world, how you develop it, and how it is received. When you give to the community, your gift is respect and admiration. This in turn builds your reputation and attracts opportunities to you. This section can be enhanced with the following:

- Green and red color hues
- Groupings of three representing the triangular shape of the flame
- Star, diamond, pointy and pyramid shapes
- Candles, bright lighting or images of the sun
- Diplomas, awards or any accolades received
- Ancient mystical symbol of the "eye" as it denotes illumination
- Images of how you want to be known in the outside world

- Physical symbol of your future goal
- Symbols of success
- Affirmations about self-respect and respect of others

<u>Enhancing Elements:</u> Wood and Fire
<u>Detrimental Elements:</u> Water, Metal, Earth

<u>Kun (2) Relationships & Commitment:</u> This gua is located to the far right corner upon door entry or between (202.5-247.5) compass points. The ch'i in this area represents the ultimate yin and receptive earth energy. It is about learning how to develop trust, openness, and an unconditional commitment to another. The element of two coming together with mutual support and love, assures happiness. This section can be enhanced with the following:

- Fire and earth color hues
- Photos of you and a significant other
- Flowers especially roses
- Romantic symbols and images (hearts, love knot, two cranes that mate for life)
- Rose quartz heart crystals
- Wedding album or honeymoon photos
- Anything that represents love and romance to you
- Romantic artwork scenes
- Sleep with your head pointed to your romance direction (see chapt. 7)
- Plant two fruit trees in your yard
- Place two candles in this sector in your bedroom to spark romance
- Affirmations to attract love and committed relationships in your life

<u>Enhancing Elements:</u> Earth and Fire
<u>Detrimental Elements:</u> Metal, Water, Wood

<u>Dui (7) Creativity & Children:</u> This gua is located in the middle one-third of the right wall upon door entry or between (247.5-292.5) compass points. This ch'i represents a childlike joyful energy. It is the part of you that yearns to explore, be free, playful, and creative. This is where you can let go of your inhibitions and let your inner child run wild. To really understand this sector, observe a child at play and notice the sheer joy that consumes them. This is the key to the type of ch'i expression here. To enhance this section any of the following can be used.

- Metals, white and pastel colors
- Any creative objects, art supplies or projects in progress
- Pictures of children
- Children's toys or art projects done by them
- Metal objects
- Oval, round or arched shapes
- Hobby items, stereos, CD's
- Fresh blooming flowers preferably white
- Baby items if you are planning on having a child
- Any goals that require creative vision
- Great area for a child's bedroom
- Affirmations confirming your creative nature and inner child

Enhancing Elements: Metal and Earth
Detrimental Elements: Water, Wood, Fire

Qian (6) Helpful People & Travel: This gua is located in the near right one-third of the front wall or between (292.5-337.5) compass points. This ch'i energy is about strength, tenacity, inspiration, and confidence. There is a responsible leadership quality that emanates from this life station and a universal life force of support. When you are in direct alignment with your soul's mission, you attract helpful people into your life and are able to manifest your destiny. You can enhance this section with any of the following items.

- Earth and metal color hues
- Pictures of mentors or people assisting others
- Images of guardian angels or saints to call upon
- Objects of travel or places you would like to go
- Metal elements
- Round, oval and arched shapes
- Movement device to call helpful people into your life
- Affirmations to draw helpful people into your life or your travel dream destination

Enhancing Elements: Metal and Earth
Detrimental Elements: Water, Wood, Fire

Kan (1) Career: This gua is located in the middle one-third of the front wall upon door entry or between (337.5-22.5) compass points. This section represents the beginning of your life's work. Like the deep waters of the ocean and quiet of the mid-winter, this sector challenges you throughout life forcing you to delve deep into your being and learn what you feel you can accomplish in this world. You can enhance this section with any of the following items.

- Deep blue and black colors
- Water features such as aquariums, fountains or water scenes
- Powerful images such as buildings, bridges or mountains
- Wavy or irregular shapes and patterns
- Career images, business cards or logos
- Hang wind chimes (outdoors only) to attract more opportunities to you
- Bird feeder or birdbath to attract life force energy here
- Healthy plant to symbolize career growth
- Affirmation to reinforce your life's mission and joy in your work

Enhancing Elements: Water and Metal
Detrimental Elements: Wood, Fire, Earth

Gen (8) Self Cultivation & Knowledge: This gua is located to the near left one-third of the front wall or between (22.5-67.5) compass degree points. The ch'i here represents a calm stillness of the mountain energy. The stillness of the mountain holds great wisdom and knowledge internally and, comparatively when you are able to quiet your mind, you become aware of this wisdom and knowledge yourself. Meditation and introspective thinking is the essence of true knowledge and will give you the strength and tenacity to walk through life. To enhance this section any of the following items can be used.

- Fire and earth color hues
- Books or study materials
- Meditation tapes, CD's or books
- Books on self-help or self-cultivation
- Pictures of people who are known for great wisdom
- A globe in this area enhances knowledge of the world
- Images of mountains will enhance this quiet ch'i
- Earth elements

- Square or rectangular shapes and patterns
- Movement device to encourage the flow of knowledge
- Affirmations regarding knowledge and inner growth

<u>Enhancing Elements:</u> Earth and Fire
<u>Detrimental Elements:</u> Metal, Water, Wood

<u>Center:</u> The center is the central point and stabilizer for the other eight guas. It is a neutral point in terms of polarity and is an extremely powerful point overall. There is no trigram for this sector, but it shares the elemental qualities of Kun and Gen (Earth sectors). This area represents YOU and vibrates to your subconscious mind. Therefore, it is important to reach within and determine what it is you truly want in life, or what brings you sheer joy. To enhance this sector any of the following items can be used.

- Yellow hues
- Keep the area clean and free of clutter
- Earth elements including terra cotta, ceramics and stone sculptures
- Square or rectangular shapes and patterns
- A great place for a meditation area
- Flowers or vital plant suggesting health and vitality for the overall body and system
- Affirmations confirming overall health and stability in life

<u>Enhancing Elements:</u> Fire and Earth
<u>Detrimental Elements:</u> Metal, Water, Wood

These are the guas represented on a symbolic level. The images, sounds, colors, and textures you surround yourself with are an integral component to your overall health, vitality, and success in life. Taking the time to assess your space to determine if it nurtures you, or if it represents your goals and life aspirations is worth the effort. Remember, you are an extension of your environment, so treat it as you would treat your own body.

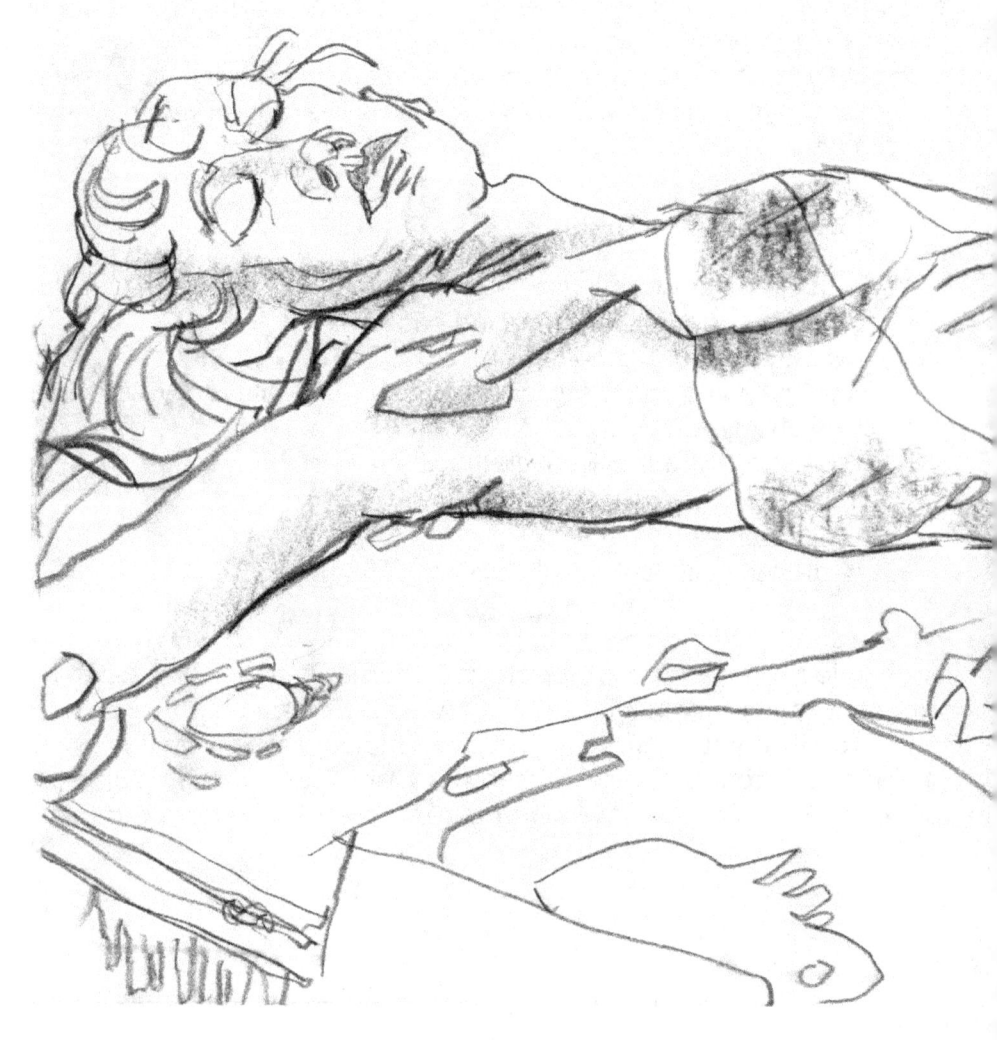

"The art of life lies in a constant readjustment to our surroundings."

Okakura Kakuzo

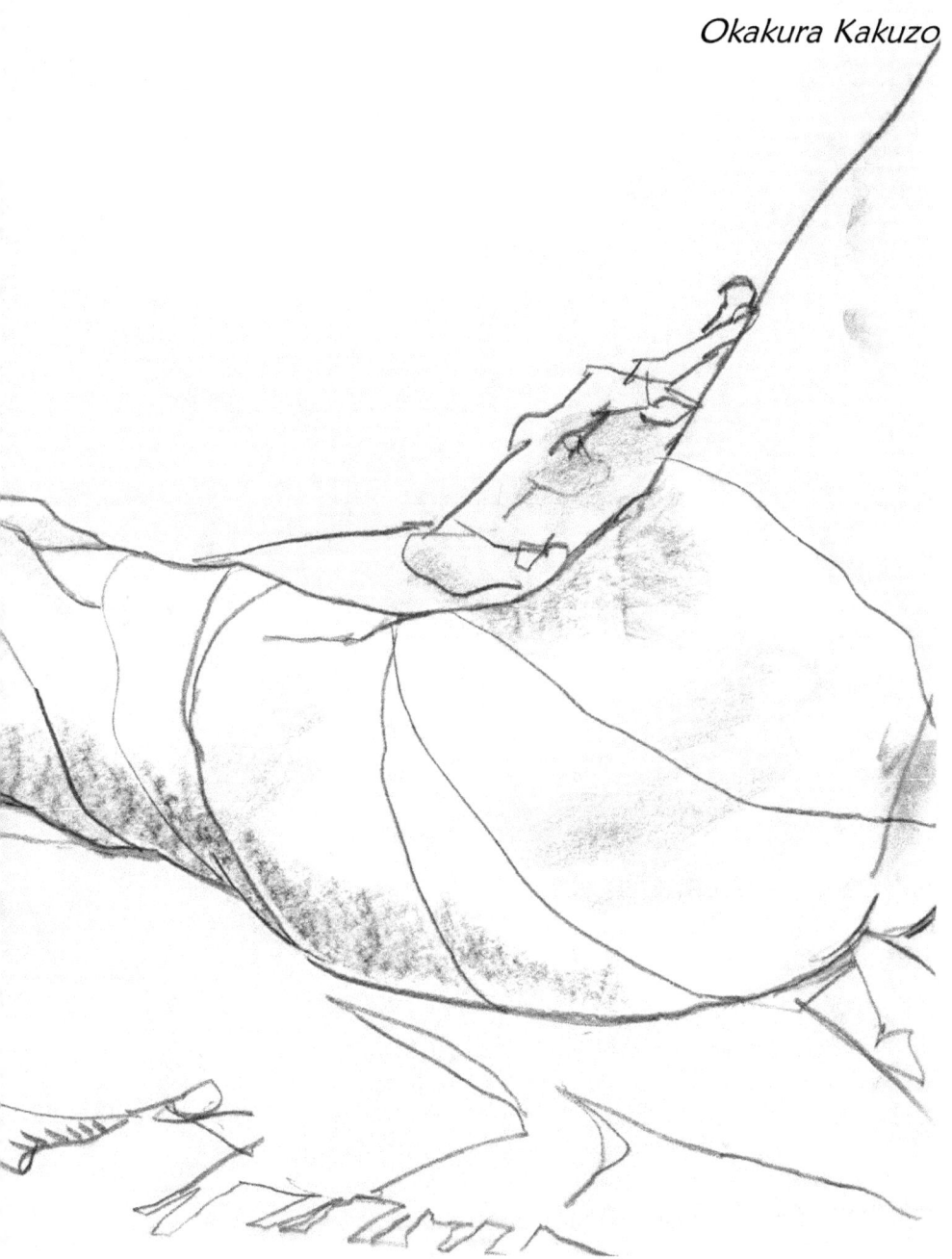

7

Designing The Essential Rooms For Health

"In dwelling, live close to the ground."

Tao Te Ching

Circulating ch'i within your environment has a profound impact on your personal ch'i vibration and ultimately determines your well-being. Therefore, it behooves you to make informed decisions when it comes to building and designing your spaces. I can't stress this point enough, as we all begin with ch'i from the same initial source – the cosmos. This ch'i is a result of minute particles that descend into the earth's atmosphere due to the planets rotating around the ecliptic band. The ch'i then filters into countries, states, towns, and finally into your home where it is imbued by the building materials, architectural shape, and finally your personal objects.

One of the best ways to align your own personal ch'i with that of your home is to work with your good directional points. In compass school feng shui, this is known as the East/West formula, or eight-house system. This theory operates under the premise that the eight cardinal directions hold a unique ch'i energy that is either positive or negative to an individual. The formula divides the eight trigrams of the ba-gua (Zhen, Xun, Li, Kun, Dui, Qian, Kan, Gen) into two groups (east & west).

East Group:		West Group	
Trigram	Direction	Trigram	Direction
Zhen: Thunder	East	Qian: Heaven	Northwest
Xun: Wind	Southeast	Dui: Lake	West
Li: Fire	South	Gen: Mountain	Northeast
Kan: Water	North	Kun: Earth	Southwest

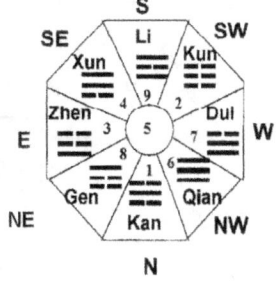

Fig. 31

Bagua

When using this formula, you can determine which group you belong to and, as a result, find out those directions that align to your personal ch'i in a positive aspect, along with those directions that have a negative impact on you. If you belong to an east group, all four of the associated directions are favorable for you, whereas the directions for the west group are unfavorable. If you refer to chapter 3, "Birth Trigram Calculation," the steps were given on how to determine your personal Ming Kua number. In that chapter we examined the traits associated with the personal trigram or Ming Kua. In this section, we will use that same number to determine the auspicious and inauspicious directions associated with that trigram. For example, if the Ming Kua was calculated to be a 3, the personal trigram that corresponds to this number is Zhen. This trigram relates to thunder and the east direction on the ba-gua. If you refer to figure 31, Zhen belongs to the east group and the associated directions are south, southeast, north, and east; The problematic directions are southwest, northeast, northwest, and west. Below is a convenient chart depicting the kua numbers and their associated groups with directional influences.

	East Group				West Group			
Kua #	3	4	1	9	6	2	8	7
1	S	N	SE	E	W	NE	SW	NW
2	SE	E	S	N	SW	NW	W	NE
3	N	S	E	SE	NE	W	NW	SW
4	E	SE	N	S	NW	SW	NE	W
P-1	SW	NW	W	NE	SE	E	S	N
P-2	NE	W	NW	SW	N	S	E	SE
P-3	NW	SW	NE	W	E	SE	N	S
P-4	W	NE	SW	NW	S	N	SE	E

1 - Prosperity	P-1 Arguments
2 - Romantic Relationships	P-2 Failed Relationships
3 - Good Health	P-3 Accidents
4 - Peace & Stability	P-4 Misfortune

* P stands for problematic   Fig. 32

Designing The Essential Rooms For Health

These directions can now be used to set up rooms appropriate for the ch'i associated with them, or simply to align the most important rooms and areas that have the greatest impact on your health. These rooms and areas consist of the bedroom, kitchen, home office, and front door.

The second part of this formula, the Zhai Kua aligns the entire house with your personal ch'i. Essentially, the group a house falls into is based on its sitting compass direction (opposite how it faces). To determine the sitting compass direction, take a compass reading from your front door or facing direction and look directly opposite of that direction to determine your sitting direction. For example, if you stand at your front door or facing direction with your back towards it while you look out towards the street and note the compass direction reading (let's say 90 degrees east), then your sitting direction is exactly 180 degrees opposite (270 degrees west). It is important to make sure that you do not wear anything metal or stand near metal (this includes cars and telephone poles), because the compass reading will be compromised. In addition, make sure you have determined the correct facing point of your house by noting the open area in front. Some homes have a front door to the side that actually faces the wall of a neighbor's house, or some kind of an obstruction. In this case, your facing direction may be the window that faces the street or open yard. Once you have determined your Zhai Kua or house group, compare it to your personal Ming Kua number. The key is to choose a house that falls in your same group. The chart below is an easy reference guide to locate your house group.

Sitting Position	Facing Position	House Trigram	Element	East/West Group
S	N	Li	Fire	East
SW	NE	Kun	Earth	West
W	E	Dui	Metal	West
NW	SE	Qian	Metal	West
N	S	Kan	Water	East
NE	SW	Gen	Earth	West
E	W	Zhen	Wood	East
SE	NW	Xun	Wood	East

Fig.33

House Groups & Trigrams

Clutter

Before you can design your space for health, you must examine the issues of clutter. Clutter is the major source behind stagnation in your life. It is a symptom of what is going on in your life and the subconscious mind's way of avoiding what needs to be done. It has a tendency to throw you off track in life, question your direction, and to trigger generalized feelings of malaise.

There are many reasons why people accumulate clutter. Many times it is simply a parental influence where one or both parents had tendencies to hoard things. Other times it is simply fear of not being able to provide for one reason or another. Sometimes clutter is used as a protective barrier from fear of the unknown. Whatever the reason, clutter stagnates the life force energy (ch'i), and depending where the clutter is located in the home, according to the ba-gua, it will stifle that life area and body system. If the clutter is removed and the area is cleansed, only then will proper ch'i movement be restored.

In order to get a handle on clutter in your space, it is best to understand exactly what it is. By and large, clutter can be broken down into four categories:

- Items you do not use or like
- Unorganized items
- Too many items in a small area
- Anything unfinished physically, mentally, and spiritually

Beginning with the first category, "Items you do not use or like," are things you may have bought and no longer need, or items given to you from a family member, friend, or ex-lover, and never liked in the first place. The objects and symbols in your space are an extension of yourself. Holding onto or displaying items you dislike or no longer have any use for is like holding onto a diseased part of ourselves. Why would you want to do that?

The second category, "Unorganized items," contributes to clutter and chaos. It can cause a lack of focus, and as a result, can derail you from your intended goals. Your days are less productive because you are spending a good portion of them trying to locate items you may need. It triggers spending since you will think you need to buy certain things, when the reality is you already have them. Any way you slice it, unorganized areas are counter productive for you on every level.

The third category, "Too many things in too small a space," is a perfect example of people moving into smaller spaces from larger ones, and bringing all their possessions with them. This is commonly seen after a divorce or separation between people. This should be a time for beginning a fresh start rather than dragging the past along with you. By eliminating these items you will increase the amount of living space while cleansing painful memories. Another reason for having too many items in a small space is that sometimes people buy furniture that is inappropriate for the intended area. I always tell my clients to buy and decorate according to the size of their space to avoid this problem.

The fourth category, "Anything unfinished physically, mentally or spiritually," weighs on your mind on a daily basis and becomes stressful. It is a constant reminder of your unfinished business. The best approach is to write down one thing you will accomplish each day and physically cross it off your list. Reward yourself for a job well done, and before you know it you will have completed your goals, lifting the burden from your mind.

When analyzing the location of clutter, you will find there are specific trigger points within the home that will attract it. Areas such as dark corners, alcoves, behind doors, under stairwells, and areas in your peripheral vision, all tend to attract clutter. These areas are prone to clutter because the energy is low. The key is to boost the ch'i with bright lighting, moving objects, essential oils or crystals. Try to avoid using these areas for storage, since it will only further stagnate the ch'i. If there are space constraints and you need to store items beneath a stairwell, store them in natural containers (wicker) and place a bowl of sea salt or Epsom salt mixed with a few drops of citrus essential oils. This will entice ch'i to flow freely. Avoid, however, storing items behind doors, as this will limit the ability for the door to open fully and impact the amount of ch'i that can flow into the room.

How Clutter Affects Your Life Aspirations & Health

When superimposing the ba-gua over the entire home or an individual room via door entry or compass points, you can determine the life aspiration groups and body systems. Clutter in any gua can impact your health and livelihood negatively. Below is an overview of the type of impact clutter will have on your life.

1. <u>Family Sector:</u> Clutter in this sector can cause discord between family members and potential ailments with the liver, gallbladder, and feet.
2. <u>Wealth Sector:</u> Stagnation of your finances and resources can occur when clutter is in this section. It may also affect your thighs, waist area, liver, hips or gallbladder.
3. <u>Fame:</u> Clutter in this sector can affect how you are recognized socially and how enthusiastic you are in life. The body systems that may be affected are the eyes, heart, circulatory system, and small intestines.
4. <u>Relationship Sector:</u> Clutter in this sector can stagnate your personal and social relationships. It may cause ailments in the abdominal region or cause digestive problems.
5. <u>Creativity & Children Sector:</u> Clutter in this area can inhibit your creative juices and your ability to connect with your children or younger people. It may cause dental problems, skin irritations, or intestinal ailments.
6. <u>Helpful People Sector:</u> Clutter here can interfere with your ability to attract others into our lives for guidance. It can also hinder your desire to travel and experience the world. Headaches or chest colds can potentially occur.
7. <u>Career:</u> Clutter here tends to stagnate your career or make your job feel challenging at every turn. The urinary system and ears are the body systems that can be vulnerable to ailments.
8. <u>Knowledge & Self-Cultivation:</u> Learning may be challenging when clutter is in this sector. You may also find it difficult to grow spiritually and make clear decisions. The hands and fingers are the body parts that may experience difficulties due to stagnant ch'i from clutter build up.
9. <u>Center:</u> Clutter in the center of a room or the entire structure can cause a number of health challenges and overall feelings of confusion and instability.

In order to reach optimum health from the feng shui perspective, removal of all clutter is essential. By eliminating clutter you will feel empowered, move through life more efficiently, think more clearly, save money, opportunities will become more evident, you will feel more comfortable in your space while creating extra room, and you will feel more energetic. The key to removing clutter is to commit to removing it and to have a plan of action.

De-cluttering Plan

The easiest way to go about de-cluttering your space is to make an assessment of where it is and why it is there. Next, take several boxes or large bags and label them as follows:

- Things to keep
- Trash
- Need repair
- Items to return
- Donate
- Gift

Your bedroom or entranceway should be addressed first; otherwise, start in the area that represents a life aspiration or body system that is challenging you. If there are many areas to tackle, map out a plan of your intentions for the job and include other family members in the process, especially if they are the cause of the clutter. Begin by assessing the items in the space and note which box or bag they belong in (things to keep, trash, etc.). Avoid the temptation to transfer the clutter from one room to another. Many times areas such as the attic or basement become "drop zones" because they are positioned out of plain view. Clutter in the attic places pressure above you stifling our future goals, while clutter in the basement can keep you from moving forward in life. Take your time during the process and take periodic breaks to avoid stress. Photograph your progress, space clear your newly organized area (see chapter 8), and reward yourself for a job well done!

The de-cluttering process within the home symbolically represents a cleansing of the body, so this is a perfect time to make adjustments in your diet and exercise routine. Maintain the momentum by staying committed to the process. Stay on top of daily mail, paperwork, laundry, recycling bins, the kitchen and bathrooms. Walk through your home from a visitor's perspective and take note of anything that looks problematic. Burn incense and spray essential oils to refresh and uplift the ch'i daily. Once your place is in order, than you can begin to implement feng shui cures and designs.

The Front Yard

The front yard is your first chance to transmute the incoming ch'i, especially from those homes adjacent to yours. In other words, if your neighbor's property is unkempt, then the ch'i that enters your property is compromised. In order to counteract this problematic ch'i from entering your personal space, it is imperative your property looks auspicious. The following is a curbside appeal checklist that will transpose unhealthy ch'i to healthy ch'i.

Curbside Appeal Checklist

- Well-groomed lawn
- Curved pathways that are well lit
- Distinct direction to front door
- Trimmed vegetation
- Nothing blocking pathways, windows, or doors
- Varying heights in vegetation
- Colorful flowers
- Year round vegetation (Arborvitaes, Evergreens, Boxwoods, etc.)
- Water feature in front to cultivate abundant ch'i
- Attract life force with bird feeder or birdbath
- Movement objects such as chimes, flags, wind socks or whirly-gigs to circulate ch'i
- Balance of yin and yang (shade & sun)
- Driveway and pathways are in good repair with no cracks

The Front Door

The front door is one of the most important features in feng shui and if well positioned will encourage health, wealth, and a long life. The main entrance is subject to the heaviest traffic flow and therefore will paint your own personal ch'i every time you pass through it.

In feng shui, the main door entrance should always be proportionate to the size of the house. If it is overly large, ch'i can leak out and can cause the occupants financial strain leading to stress and compromised health. On the flip side, if the door is overly small in relation to the house size, then ch'i is squelched causing an array of challenges from bickering to having to work harder than usual for everything in life. Below is the front door checklist that will attract beneficial ch'i.

Front Door Checklist

- Welcoming and well maintained presentation with fresh paint
- Shiny features such as address numbers, knocker, or kick plate
- Wood door will provide stability and protection
- Fully functional with no hindrances
- Decorative wreath, plaque, or family crest
- Large chime positioned at least 4 feet from the door to attract ch'i
- Curved (half moon) welcome mat
- Avoid poor alignment with trees, poles, T-junction, Y-junction, Dead End, bladed curve, neighbor's driveway or garage, places of worship, cemeteries, garbage dump, police or fire station, hospital, factory, high tension wires, cell towers, large building, or a mountain
- Lighting on either side of the door to elevate ch'i and for protection
- Straight and rot free doorframes; These are the supporting poles for the family
- Preferably facing one of your auspicious directions

The Front Entrance

Your first impression is set the moment you walk through your front door. What is seen will set the tone for the ch'i in the entire home and your own personal ch'i vibration. An entranceway that is in order, clutter free, well lit, pleasant smelling, has soothing sounds, is freshly painted, and has a focal point of either a healthy plant, vase of flowers, or a beautiful sculpture, will feel welcoming and imbue the incoming ch'i with positive energy.

How the front entrance is aligned to doorways (front to back) and walls, as well as its size and height, will also impact the incoming ch'i. As previously mentioned in chapter 5, front entrances that align to back doors or windows will cause the ch'i to accelerate moving directly back out of the home. In essence, the ch'i doesn't have a chance to grace the home and feed the life areas or body meridians. The narrow entranceway constricts ch'i and the human aura causing possible respiratory ailments and anxiety. An overly high foyer ceiling causes the ch'i to flow upwards minimizing the amount of ch'i source in the immediate area. Any hindrance in the architecture here, such as a wall opposite the front door sets up barriers and feelings of being overwhelmed. Finally, the front entrance that opens to a staircase will cause the incoming ch'i to be sucked up to the second level and, as a result, the ch'i flow is interrupted causing ch'i from the second level to rush out of the home. Proper feng shui design for the front entrance is crucial to initiate positive ch'i flow. Below is a checklist to assist you with good entranceway feng shui.

Entranceway Checklist

- Bright lighting source
- Free of clutter
- Proper closet space for shoes, coats, hats, etc.
- Focal point of interest
- Soothing sounds and scents
- Variety of shapes, colors, finishes, and textures to create playful ch'i
- Runner, chandelier, faceted crystal, artwork, and plants when entrance opens to back door, window, or staircase
- Upward lighting & plants, light colored walls when entranceway opens from below street level (city apartment or basement apartment)

Designing The Essential Rooms For Health

<u>The Bedroom</u>

The bedroom is considered one of the most important rooms in feng shui because of its powerful impact on your health and relationships. This is a room where one third of your life is spent in a sleeping state. It is in this room that your body looks to unwind, relax, and be intimate. Poor feng shui design can cause ill health and an empty relationship. Therefore, it is paramount you look at this room with a discerning eye. Below are guidelines to follow when choosing and designing this space.

Direction: One of the most powerful energetic choices you can make regarding bedroom placement is choosing a complimentary direction to your personal Ming Kua number. By doing this, you are aligning your own personal ch'i with that of directional compatibility. If you share this room with another person from the opposite group (East/West), then a compromise needs to be made. For example, if the house (Zhai Kua) favors one person, then allow the bedroom to favor the other. However, if one person has health challenges, then choose the room direction to match that individual. Finally, many times in feng shui we will align the favorable direction to the breadwinner in the family.

If the architectural layout does not allow for the bedroom position to fall within any of the four auspicious directions, then aligning the bed (top of head points to this direction) to one of the four good directions is recommended. It is preferable to align this part of the bed with the direction for peace and stability. There is only one exception to this rule, and that is if your peaceful direction is south. In this scenario, the electromagnetic flow of the earth's magnetic field is in direct opposition to this direction. The magnetic field flows out of the North Pole around and back into the South Pole. If you are positioned with your head pointed to the south direction, ch'i will push upward against your feet and to the chest area potentially causing anxiety and abdominal ailments. Over time this reverse ch'i flow can cause the magnetic field of the body to flip.

Room Positions: Try to avoid using a room that extends beyond the alignment of the front door or other portions of the house front as your master bedroom. The extended position (from an L-shape or U-shape structure) leaves the body detached from the rest of the structure and as a result you may feel unstable and isolated. Furthermore, it is more difficult for ch'i to circulate and reach this part of the home. If you find yourself in such a scenario, the best solution is to place a beautiful vista on the shared internal wall that will create the illusion of drawing the room back in alignment with the rest of the home. You may carry a continuous design between the bedroom as well as other rooms within the main architecture of the home to symbolically draw the rooms together.

You also want to avoid bedrooms positioned above a garage or those abut a garage. In feng shui, a garage is not a supportive room and therefore will compromise the stability of the bedroom. In addition, garages tend to house toxic agents such as paints, gasoline, oil, cleaning agents, and other problematic items. These chemicals will outgas directly into the bedroom and can compromise your health. If you have no choice in the matter and must sleep above the garage, then remove all toxic chemicals, allow your car to outgas up to two hours prior to pulling into the garage, and ground the bedroom by forming a grid with stones in the four corners.

If the room abuts the garage, follow all the aforementioned solutions. Make certain there are no chemicals or sharp tools on the wall that abuts the garage. You can also place ¼ inch cork boards on the abutment wall in the garage to act as a buffer to the bedroom. This will help to insulate the problematic energy.

Bedrooms that are located beneath a bathroom, abut a kitchen, at the top of a staircase, at the end of a long hallway, in a basement or below an entrance level, all require feng shui remedies. The bedroom beneath a bathroom needs to be stabilized by placing terminating crystal points facing upwards in the four corners of the room. In the bathroom that is above the bedroom, place four stones in the corners to stabilize the constant water movement in this room.

When the bedroom abuts a kitchen, the fire element of the kitchen (yang) throws off the yin energy of the bedroom and can cause arguments, high blood pressure, and other cardiovascular issues. It is best to reposition the bed from the shared kitchen wall and place an earthy scene on that wall in the bedroom to drain the fire element of the kitchen.

When the bedroom is located at the top of a staircase that is aligned with the front door, the ch'i can be overwhelming. It is best to redirect the ch'i from the entry point of the home with a plant, decorative area rug, crystal chandelier, faceted crystal or artwork, and always keep the bedroom door closed at night.

If a bedroom is situated at the end of a long hallway the ch'i will run quickly directed towards the bed. In this case, place a decorative floor runner, a faceted crystal, or stagger artwork along the hallway walls to slow the ch'i movement. In addition, keep the bedroom door closed at night.

Finally, bedrooms that are located in a basement or below an entrance level have poor ch'i circulation and quality. These rooms usually have lower ceilings and smaller windows, if any. Incorporate incandescent upward lighting, romantic artwork with upward movement, a plant or salt lamp to purify the air, terminating crystal points, and use lighter color hues. These remedies will help to uplift the otherwise suppressive ch'i.

Bed Placement: The placement of the bed is one of the most important interior design factors when it comes to feng shui and good health. It is best to place the bed on a solid wall facing the door entrance (mouth of incoming ch'i). This alignment places the body in a command position keeping it in a relaxed state. The command position is best when the bed is located diagonally to the door entrance. This position avoids a direct onslaught of ch'i bombarding the foot of the bed and causing potential foot problems. Because of this, it is important that you do not align the bed directly to the doorway entrance. This is known as the coffin or mortuary position in feng shui and considered inauspicious.

When positioning the bed, it is best to place it on an interior solid wall as oppose to under a window or exterior wall. The body will feel more grounded in this position and maintain a high energy level. If there are architectural constraints leaving you no other choice but to place the bed beneath a window, then a protective barrier such as heavy drapery, solid headboard, or euro-pillows will buffer the otherwise unsupportive feature. Placing a rose quartz stone beneath the head of the mattress will also relax the body in this position.

Try to avoid placing the bed beneath overhead beams. The right angles created between the beam and ceiling cause a back flow of ch'i resulting in downward pelting energy at approximately 96 feet per second. This is extremely stressful for the body over an eight-hour sleeping period. If you have no other choice, you can paint the beams the same color as the ceiling or install decorative brackets where the beams meet the wall. Any of these remedies will capture the ch'i from being directed to the bed and hitting the body. A bed positioned beneath a sloping ceiling is also problematic, as the ch'i is extremely oppressive and restrictive. Once again, it is best to reposition the bed, but if you are unable to do so, then place terminating crystal points facing upward toward the ceiling along with incandescent lighting projected upward. These remedies will help to uplift the otherwise suppressive ch'i.

Avoid placing a bed where it crosses the bedroom door, as the ch'i will cut directly across the bed disrupting sleep and causing pain in the area of the body in direct alignment to this path. The best remedy is to reposition the bed. If you are unable to do so, the easiest solution is to keep the door closed at night.

Placing a bed cattycorner in a room is also problematic, as the ch'i tends to swirl behind the head and can potentially cause headaches. If this position is unable to change, then try to soften the ch'i by placing a decorative curtain behind the bed to absorb the swirling ch'i.

Finally, avoid placing the bed on a wall that has electrical equipment, appliances, or a hot water heater. These objects emit EMF's that are not diminished by walls. A safe distance is at least three yards away from these sources. If the bed shares the wall of these appliances, the likelihood is you will not be protected. This position may cause anxiety, insomnia, headaches, arguments, allergies, and other ailments. In this scenario, it is best to reposition the bed and place resonator tabs on the appliances (see resource section).

Furniture: Bedroom furniture should be made with natural materials that can breathe. This is healthiest for the body, especially when it comes to the bed itself. Try to avoid synthetic materials such as Formica, laminates or lacquer furniture. These materials outgas and can have a negative impact on your health and can potentially cause allergies and headaches. The headboard should be well constructed and firmly attached to the bed. This will provide support for the head and aid in sound sleep. Try to avoid four posted beds with heavy wood and canopies, as they will feel claustrophobic.

When arranging bedroom furniture, try to be cognizant of positioning large pieces too close to the bed. The body will have difficulty relaxing because of the potential injury that could be inflicted if the piece topples over. Also, be aware of any right angles or poison arrows directed towards the bed from the furniture. The best way to determine whether furniture is projecting a poison arrow or spiraling ch'i is to lie in the bed and take note of any sharp corners directed towards the bed. If you find there are sharp corners, then assess which part of the body is in alignment with them. Since ch'i cannot fully navigate a right angle, the energy will continue to move forward spiraling at full speed until something in its path absorbs it. If that something happens to be your body, then over time you may experience pain in that particular area. The best solution is to reposition the furniture. However, if that is not an option, simply place something between you and the furniture to absorb the spiraling ch'i. This can be a decorative throw draped over the furniture, or place a small red dot (marker, nail polish or red tape) just beneath the corner of the furniture. The red color will attract the ch'i and pull it back into itself. This is such a simple solution yet highly effective. During my feng shui classes, I demonstrate this while using a dowsing rod. It always amazes my students how the dowsing rod reacts to the red tape when placed on a corner piece.

General Design Tips For The Bedroom

Symbolism: The symbolism in this room should exude romance, relaxation, and vitality. Romantic artwork, sculptures, and symbols placed to the far right side of the room, or southwest sector will strengthen the relationship and lead to happiness and contentment with your partner. An image of vitality and strength (mountain, field of poppies, vineyard, etc.) placed in the health sector, or east direction will support your health.

Scents: Romantic scents such as Pink Grapefruit, Ylang Ylang or Jasmine sprayed daily on sheets and throughout the room will freshen ch'i and activate the olfactory gland, a very powerful mood elevator. You may also spray Lavender essential oil to calm and relax the body.

Colors: Color has a powerful impact on the human aura and chakra system and therefore can impact your mood and health. Subdued (yin) and romantic colors are appropriate for this room. Skin tone colors will nurture the body while mauve, green, burgundy and rose colors will aid in romance. The key is to choose a color hue that is subtle to relax the body, rather than colors that will excite it. Try to avoid yellow, lavender, blue, or brown in this room, as these colors are too thought provoking, chaste, cool, and structured respectively.

Window Treatment: Choose natural fabrics with a romantic color theme that provide good coverage to shield light pollution from street lamps or other outdoor night lighting. This is very important, as the body needs total darkness when sleeping for the pineal gland to reset the cascade of hormones.

Too much light source in the bedroom can interfere with restful sleep, and as a result serotonin levels can drop, affecting the hormonal system.

Remove All Work Items: Work related items are associated with yang energy; therefore, they are in direct opposition to the yin nature of this room. When these items are in plain view, it becomes difficult for the body to fully relax since there is a constant reminder to work. In addition, work items in the bedroom will put a strain on the relationship, since the focus shifts from the relationship to work.

Remove Exercise Equipment: Stationary bikes, yoga mats, abdominal rollers, or any other piece of exercise equipment represents yang energy and therefore will excite the body when it is trying to calm down and relax. This equipment should be relocated to another room so the body is not interrupted during rest. If space constraints are an issue, then screen the equipment to shield it from plain view, otherwise the body will be programmed to exercise instead of rest.

<u>Remove All Electromagnetics:</u> If you refer to chapter 4, there is extensive information regarding the detrimental effects electromagnetics have on the human body. These adverse effects are exacerbated during sleep since the body is in an extremely vulnerable state. The two most common appliances people have difficulty parting with are digital clock radios and televisions. If you refuse to part with these items, at the very least encase the television inside an armoire and disconnect the remote control. Furthermore, remove the clock radio from the nightstand and place it on a dresser at least six feet from the bed. Although this may seem like an inconvenience, you will be creating a healthier sleeping environment for yourself.

<u>Remove Clutter:</u> Clutter stagnates ch'i and depending where it is located in the ba-gua map of the room, it can stagnate that part of your life and body system. Anything that you dislike, no longer have use for, or is broken needs to be removed from the room, especially if any of these items are stored beneath the bed. The bed should never be compromised in any manner, as ch'i needs to circulate freely beneath it.

<u>Linens:</u> The bedroom is a place where you begin and end your day. Therefore, if there were any room to indulge yourself in, this would be it. Choose soothing linens with natural fibers to minimize the static electric charge. Also, add an element of romance such as chenille and silk. Ensconce yourself in these luxurious fabrics and enjoy this part of your day to relax and romance.

The Home Office

More and more people are working from home making this room one of the top four important rooms in feng shui. Since a home office has contact with the outside world, it is best to position it in the yang side (front) of the home. However, this is an ideal opportunity to locate the office in your personal Ming Kua direction for success. If that is not feasible, then aligning your desk to face your prosperity point is also very auspicious. It is extremely important however that you do not compromise your command position to the door in order to align your desk to this directional point. Command always takes precedence over any other factors, since it will keep the body in a calm state.

Below are guidelines for designing a healthy office.

Healthy Office Design

- Command the door with desk placement
- Use a wooden desk (natural materials)
- Place several plants in the office to purify air and absorb EMF's from equipment (peace lilies, spider, ivy)
- Decorate on the yang side
- Yellow is a great color for thinking while orange, turquoise, teal and blue are great colors for creativity
- Use appropriate symbolism pertaining to career including nameplate, business cards, brochures, etc.
- Have sufficient filing systems
- Place a water feature in the north sector or southeast sector of the office
- Incorporate movement devices to circulate ch'i
- Place natural quartz crystals near computer to absorb EMF's
- Incorporate a salt lamp to increase the amount of negative ions in the air
- Use an incandescent lighting source
- Avoid right angles (poison arrows) projected to work area; Soften with draping plants if need be
- If outside clients visit the office, then it is best to have a separate entrance
- Make sure the desk is supported by a solid wall
- Use EMF tabs on copy machines, CPU's and computer monitors (see resource section)
- Avoid sitting under beams and sloping ceilings
- Avoid clutter including in the hard drive
- Spray essential oils daily
- Avoid commingling the work area with personal living space
- Keep ergonomics in mind to avoid stress

Kitchen

The kitchen is the final room of the top four areas (front door, bedroom, home office, kitchen) that have the greatest impact on your health and livelihood. In feng shui, the kitchen represents your health (how I feed myself) and prosperity (the ability to feed myself). The most auspicious location for a kitchen is in the southern, southeastern or eastern side of the home. These directions are in harmony with the fire elemental quality of this room. For example, the south direction on the ba-gua map represents the fire element, and the east and southeast directions correspond to the wood element. In five element theory, the wood element feeds the fire source making this element very beneficial for this room. Furthermore, prior to gas or electric cooking devices, wood was used to create the fire for cooking.

If your kitchen is located in another direction, simply balance it by using five-element theory (chapter 3) to keep the fire element strong. For example, if the kitchen is located in the northeast, the earth element of this direction will naturally deplete the fire element of the kitchen. In this scenario, simply place more wood elements to support the fire and uproot the earth.

As previously mentioned in chapter five, the kitchen should be well protected and not visible from the front entrance. You should have a full view of the room and not a partial or split view. The doorway should not be too narrow otherwise the ch'i will funnel causing negative energy. There should also be more than one door entrance into this room to ensure good ch'i circulation. It should be centrally located in the home for easy access, but not positioned through the center point of the home.

When designing this room, one of the most important elements is the placement of the stove. It is best to position the stove in a center island since the chef will be able to have full command of the kitchen. If this is not feasible due to space constraints, then placement should still give the chef at least a side command to the doorway entrance. If the design does not allow for direct or side command, then incorporate a reflective surface behind the stove to provide indirect vision for the chef. This is an important concept because having your back to the door places the body in a vulnerable position and physiologically the fight or flight mechanism is initiated causing adrenalin, cortisol, and other stress hormones to be released in the body. It is also considered very auspicious for the incoming fuel source to the stove to be aligned with one of the chef's auspicious directions. This is a traditional concept followed in China, since preparing food and nourishment is regarded as a "treasure." Below are additional kitchen design guidelines to follow.

Kitchen Design Guidelines

- Ch'i should circulate freely
- Avoid placing water features (refrigerator, sink) along side stove; These two elements (water & fire) clash
- Eliminate clutter including broken appliances, old cookware and utensils, unused gadgets, outdated food, rotting fruits and vegetables, garbage, used plastic bags, old pieces of dishware, etc.
- Avoid racks over an island, as it is too oppressive
- Paint this room in brighter colors, with the exception of reds, as this color will add too much fire source to a fire room
- Place healthy plants, herbs, vegetables, and fruits in this room; They can be presented symbolically in artwork, plaques, or bowls
- Utilize efficient storage systems and cabinetry
- Use natural building elements (ceramic, terra cotta, slate, cement, granite, wood, bamboo, wicker)
- Keep sharp utensils or cooking tools in cabinets or drawers
- Minimize what is stored on the countertops
- Make sure all stove burners work and rotate usage
- Empty garbage and recycling bins daily
- Use natural or incandescent lighting sources
- Incorporate curves
- Choose a round or oval table, as ch'i can spin freely to aid in conversation
- Keep the television out of this room, as the focus should be on the family and nourishment
- Use traditional ovens as opposed to microwaves
- Avoid bathrooms that are inside or abut a kitchen

Designing The Essential Rooms For Health

Social Rooms

Social rooms can be classified as a living room, dining room, or family room. These are spaces where family and friends gather and therefore should be situated on the ground floor. They also can be positioned in the front (yang) side of the house, since by and large entertainment is the main focus for these rooms. These rooms should be welcoming, relaxing, and designed to invoke conversation. Try to arrange couches and chairs in a circular layout and position it so command is possible. If you are unable to give command from all seats, then provide indirect command (mirror) and support (wall, screen or heavy drapery) for those seats in an otherwise vulnerable position. It is also important to arrange seating so the television is not the main focus. If that is difficult to configure, then enclose the television inside an armoire. This is a good idea anyway, as the focus should be on family and friends, not the television. Below is a list of some additional design guidelines for social rooms.

Social Rooms Feng Shui Design Guidelines

- Avoid placing seating beneath beams or sloping ceilings
- Incorporate a variety of lighting sources for different activities (bright for reading and games, lower for movies and relaxation)
- Fireplaces should be balanced with plants (wood) to feed the fire, and water (mirror, glass, fish sculptures) to keep the fire under control
- Use natural materials in furnishings and fabrics such as hard wood, wood furniture, wicker, bamboo, rattan, cotton, etc.
- Encase the television and stereo components inside an armoire
- Bring in nature's elements (plants, flowers, water features)
- Paintings and objects displayed should be pleasant, uplifting, and have a harmonious theme
- Eliminate clutter (old magazines, broken items, newspapers, toys, etc.)
- Screen off any play or work areas that are shared with this room due to space constraints
- Use softer (yin) colors to invoke relaxation
- Keep exposed bookshelves orderly and spacious
- In a dining room use lower lighting and artwork relating to health and vitality; Use an even number of chairs, an oval or round table, and incorporate natural elements and materials

- Avoid placing towering furniture along side seating areas or immediate to the left of the door entrance; It will feel threatening and block ch'i flow respectively
- Avoid sunk-in living rooms and family rooms, as the lower position pulls ch'i downward; Use up-lighters, columnar shapes, and patterns to uplift the ch'i in this scenario
- Avoid overly high ceiling designs (12-30 feet), as the ch'i is sucked upward leaving a depleted source of ch'i in the living area
- Minimize the size and number of windows in this space, otherwise you will feel exposed and vulnerable to the outside world

Bathrooms & Utility Rooms

These rooms are considered wet rooms in feng shui and synonymous with a draining energy. Although there is a lot of water in these rooms, and in feng shui water is associated with wealth, the water used in these rooms is waste water; therefore, it symbolizes the disposal of wealth. Where these rooms are located, especially the bathroom is key in terms of livelihood and your health. Try to avoid positioning the bathroom near an entrance, at the opposite end of the entrance, above an entrance, inside or near the kitchen, in the center of the home, or inside a bedroom. These positions are considered inauspicious disrupting and clashing with the ch'i dynamics of these areas. Wherever the bathroom is located, it should always be decorated lavishly, have fresh linens, natural elements including ceramic tiles, granite, slate, etc. It should also be freshly painted and incorporate plants, flowers, candles, fresh bath salts or oils, as this room is also where you cleanse your body and soul.

Remedies For Problematic Bathroom Placement

<u>Near, Above or Opposite Main Entrance:</u> When a bathroom is positioned right near the front entrance, benevolent yang ch'i entering will be attracted to the yin water of the bathroom and disposed of before it has a chance to modulate throughout the space. In this case, decorate luxuriously, keep the door closed, the toilet lid down, drains closed, and wrap red electrical tape around (3 times) where the sink basin meets the incoming water line pipe. You may also hang a decorative wreath or stone plaque on the door to shift the focus from

Designing The Essential Rooms For Health

the bathroom. The same remedies should be put into play when the bathroom is situated at the end of a long hallway opposite the front door. In addition to the aforementioned remedies, place a decorative runner, faceted crystal, and artwork staggered on the walls of the hallway to slow fast moving ch'i down. When the bathroom is positioned above an entranceway, stabilize it by placing four stones in the corners. In addition, placing a healthy plant in the bathroom will effectively drain the otherwise negative water associated with this type of wet-room. These cures will ground the instability associated with the bathroom and minimize the effects of the location above the entranceway.

<u>Bathroom Inside Kitchen or Abut Kitchen:</u> In this scenario, it is important to keep the drains closed, toilet lid down, and the door closed while positioning craft-size mirrors with the reflective side toward the bathroom. These mirrors can be placed inside cabinets or behind artwork depending on the layout design. The photonic energy from the mirrors will push the bathroom energy back to where it belongs.

<u>Bathroom Positioned in Center of Home:</u> The center point of a home is the stabilizing factor for the entire structure. This can be compared to the abdomen in the human body being the center point, or our stabilizing core. The center area of a room or building is represented by the earth element and is the only point where all the other life aspiration points of the ba-gua meet. The constant water movement in a bathroom located here will destabilize the entire structure and exhaust the earth element. To remedy this situation, incorporate earth elements (the color yellow, ceramic, terra cotta, granite, check patterns, etc.) in the bathroom to hold back the water element and support the earth element. You may also place four stones in the corners of the bathroom to ground and stabilize it, along with placing a bamboo plant to uplift the ch'i and further drain the water element.

<u>Bathroom Located in Bedroom:</u> The bathroom represents a yin energy and therefore when located within a bedroom will deplete the yang energy of the occupants. It is important to keep the drains closed, toilet lid down, and keep the door closed, especially if it is aligned with the bed. To further stabilize this energy, place grounding stones in the four corners of the bathroom.

Bathroom Located In The Guas

There is no gua that a bathroom can safely be positioned in simply because of its unstable draining effects. The best way then to counteract the draining effects, is to follow the aforementioned remedies, and then add proper symbolism and images to the bathroom according to the gua location in the overall ba-gua. For example, if the bathroom happens to fall in the relationship gua, either in the overall structure or a room, simply incorporate some romantic images to the bathroom design. If it is located in a health gua, then incorporate thriving plants or images of vitality (strong mountain, field of poppies, etc.). If the bathroom is in the fame area include fire elements in the décor. Candles are a wonderful fire element and provide a relaxing spa-like feel.

Additional Bathroom & Utility Room Design Guidelines

- Fix all leaks, as water symbolically represents wealth and translates into money down the drain
- Decorate these rooms lavishly
- Incorporate natural materials such as ceramic, terra cotta, granite, slate; They will look dynamic and also will exhaust the water element associated with these rooms
- Place vibrant plants (silk or real), as the wood element will drain the water element of these rooms and incorporate columnar shapes and patterns to uplift the overly yin ch'i
- Position the toilet out of plain view when entering the bathroom, it is undesirable
- Keep drains closed, toilet lids down, and use red electrical tape around all incoming water pipes to hold back the otherwise draining effects of the water
- Incorporate bright lighting sources (incandescent bulbs only)
- Use mirrors to enlarge small bathrooms
- Incorporate curves in bathroom and utility rooms
- Store only natural cleaning products and detergents
- Use screens to block view of a bathroom without a door in suites
- Keep bath salts and oils for relaxation and renewal
- Eliminate all clutter including outdated prescriptions, old toothbrushes or razors, old detergents, empty soap dispensers or shampoo bottles, and empty toothpaste tubes

- Empty garbage daily
- Use natural (wicker, bamboo or cotton) storage containers
- Have ample cabinetry and storage solutions
- Clean daily with natural cleaning agents
- Place wet towels in laundry
- Do laundry daily

Sacred Space

In traditional Chinese culture and Buddhist families, a room was chosen, preferably towards the center of the home, for meditation and thanksgiving. A small alter was dedicated to Buddha and ancestors of the family. This is a wonderful concept that we can all benefit from, especially in this day in age when an overabundance of activities fills our day with little time left for spiritual renewal. If your home is large enough to dedicate an entire room for this purpose, you will find it to be most beneficial for you. If not, you can use a tray to place a candle, incense stick, crystal and other items that hold deep meaning for you and take it out daily for meditative prayer.

Design this room with softer (yin) color hues. Purple in particular is the color for spirituality and meditative activities. Place images in here with deep meaning and spiritual essence. Incorporate comfortable seating or floor pillows for prayer and meditation. The lighting source should be low, or just use candles. Burn incense, waft essential oils, and incorporate sounds of nature or Zen meditation sounds. Bring in stones and crystals to ground and energize the space, along with your favorite books with spiritual content. Use this room at least twice a day (morning and night) to decompress and align the body and soul to its natural spiritual essence. This will in turn counteract the daily stresses of life and keep you well balanced and centered.

Once you have assessed your space and followed the feng shui guidelines for healthy design, you have symbolically aligned your body to a healthier energy. Follow up on page 154 for a list of feng shui cures, ch'i boosters, and color enhancers to keep handy when addressing your surroundings.

Feng Shui Adjustments

1. <u>Lighting:</u> Can uplift and expand ch'i; Upward lighting works best in suppressed areas.
2. <u>Mirrors:</u> Can enlarge a smaller space, draw positive images into a room, deflect sha ch'i, and open up missing guas. Make sure you hang mirrors high enough so you do not cut off the head or neck of the occupants in the home.
3. <u>Sound:</u> The vibrational energy that sound creates will keep ch'i moving. This can be achieved with chimes, water features, music, or noise machines with nature sounds.
4. <u>Stability Objects:</u> Objects that are heavy such as statues, pillars, rocks or mountain images all provide a stabilizing element to a space. These work especially well in guas where you feel your life is unstable.
5. <u>Life Force:</u> Adding life to the environment is a tremendous ch'i booster. Children, pets, plants, fish and flowers are all wonderful life elements and ch'i boosters.
6. <u>Movement Objects:</u> Will circulate and assist ch'i in moving freely. Some examples are: flags, whirly gigs, wind socks, chimes, mobiles, and water features.
7. <u>Color:</u> Color is an excellent adjustment to any space, relatively inexpensive, and makes an incredible difference. Here are a few colors that can have an impact on our moods and the ch'i:

- <u>Yellow, Reds, Turquoise:</u> Lifts energy
- <u>Browns:</u> Slows energy down and grounds
- <u>Pinks, Greens and Pastels:</u> Creates a light and airy effect on ch'i
- <u>Whites and Beiges:</u> Neutralizes a space
- <u>Orange, Teal and Bright Blue:</u> Enhances creativity and imagination
- <u>Purple, Violet and White:</u> Enhances spirituality and meditation
- <u>Red, Mauve, Green, Pink:</u> Enhances romantic feelings
- <u>Black, Gold, Royal Blue and Red:</u> Enhances feelings of power
- <u>Greens, Blue and Peach:</u> Calms and relaxes the body

The key ingredients behind successfully designing your space for a healthy environment is to take your time and map out each area from the shape of the room, directional location, size, and position in the ba-gua. Know the main purpose of the room, and then decide what it is you are trying to achieve. Set your intentions, and enjoy the process.

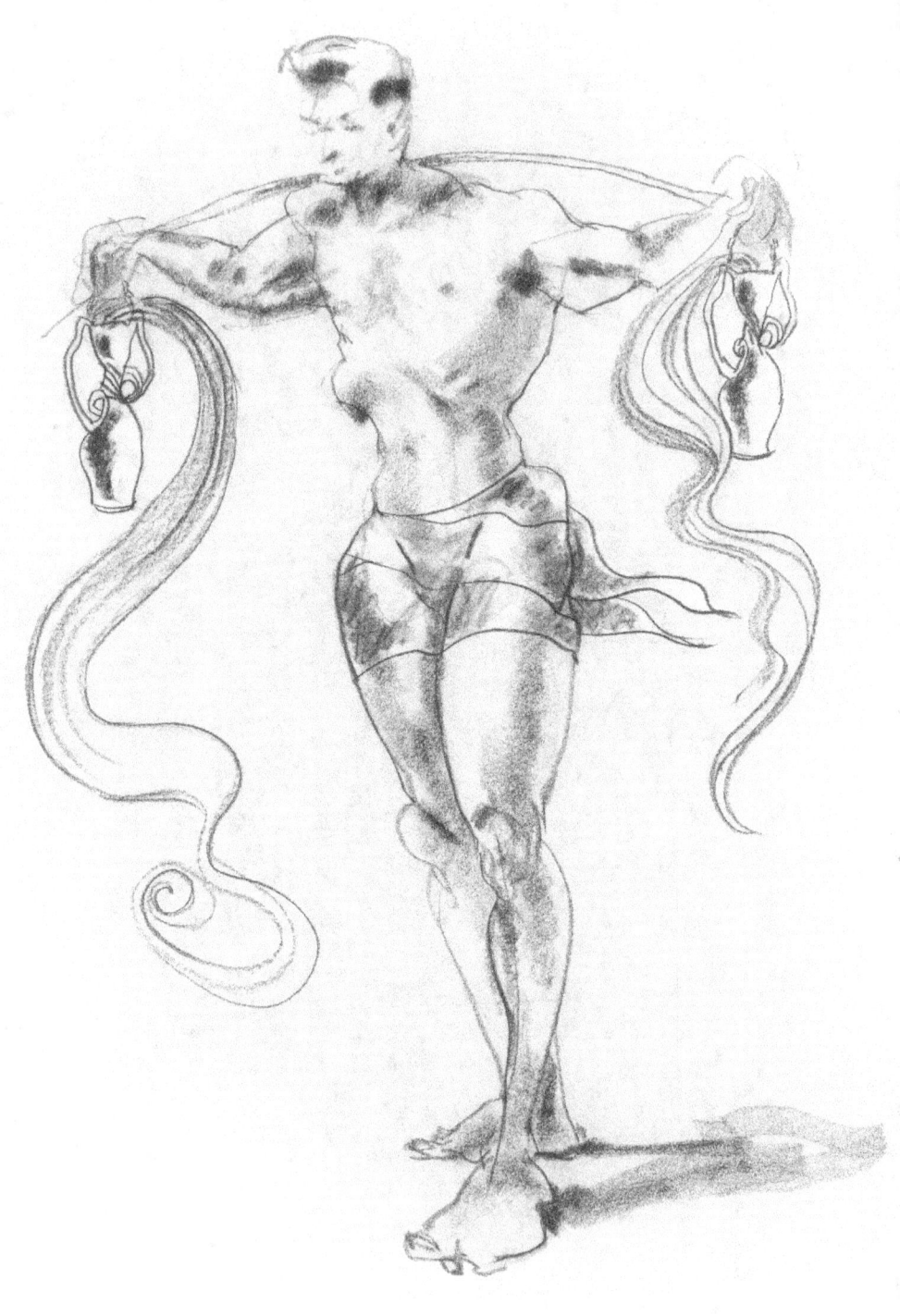

8
Consecrating Your Space

"You must give to nature more than you take. Obey it and the earth will provide you in glorious abundance."

Alan Chadwick

Historically, civilizations in China and India, as well as the Celtic tribes of England and Europe, Native American Indians, Aborginal tribes in Australia, and many others were intimately connected with nature. There was an innate wisdom and sacredness regarded for Mother Earth. These cultures recognized the importance of living in harmony with the environment and expressed it through rituals and ceremonies intended to bring about balanced energies within their dwellings. Shamans, Priests, or the holy men of the community were called upon to bless the home and remove any negative energy. In some instances these ceremonies represented humanity's age-old attempt to have a relationship with the unseen realms of life. These ceremonies conformed to the cultural traditions and particular time period in history. Even though these rituals differed from culture to culture, the underlying purpose and intention was always the same. It was all about maintaining a balanced and harmonious relationship with nature and to co-create with Mother Earth instead of having dominion over Her.

Space clearing is a sacred branch of feng shui practice that transforms our living and working spaces into sacred places. In order to understand the purpose of space clearing, it is important to know how energy is processed and how we in turn process it. Essentially, there are seven levels of energy that are contained within the atmosphere. The composition of the environment, externally and internally, determines the level of energy we are exposed to. These levels range from very low to very high. We have all experienced the impact of these levels in the way your physical, emotional, and spiritual bodies feel. For example, when you feel ill, depressed, unmotivated, or just stuck in life, it is a reflection of the energy level within your environment that you are exposed to. On the other hand, high energy levels leave you with feelings of vitality, flashes of instant knowledge, wisdom, and being more spiritually connected. Sacred places, as mentioned in chapter 4, are examples of areas that have high energy levels that can alter your physical, emotional, and spiritual state.

We are all capable of inhaling this higher energy level at anytime; unfortunately, most of us go through life in a lower level range. Space clearing is a simple way to elevate the existing energy level in your space, and in doing so, increases your own personal energy level and the ability to move through life in an awakened state. I know many of my clients report a change in how their environment feels and how they feel after a space clearing session. It is one of the easiest ways to bring about change in your life and is a wonderful accoutrement to your feng shui applications.

Building Energetics

Buildings, homes, and rooms absorb energy from any activity, disturbance, jubilation, or tragedy that occurred in them. The pattern of energy associated with the activity becomes embedded into the very fabric of the home and, as a result, these vibrations of energy become embedded within us contributing to our state of health and well-being. If we examine the energetic component of a building, there is an aura bubble that acts as a protective layer. This bubble extends around the building in two layers. The inner layer has a thickness of approximately two feet and spans outward from the building at approximately four feet in distance. The second layer is approximately three feet in depth and spans out twelve feet from the building.

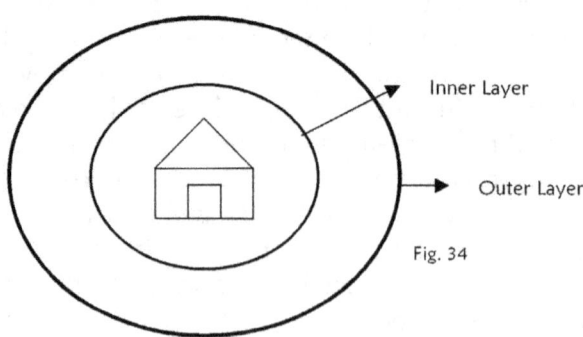

Fig. 34

Any energetic vibration from the builders, building materials, and any occupants within the structure all are stored in these two layers. Therefore, it is important to include the house aura during a space clearing ceremony.

Because your personal possessions will also lock onto energetic vibrations, it is important to assess the objects within your space and decide whether they bring energy to you or pull it away. An easy way to determine if an object is draining your energy is to walk through your home room-by-room and observe the items in the space. Notice how they make you feel. Do you smile and feel uplifted, or does it make you feel angry, disgusted, or indifferent? By decorating your space with colors, fabrics, furniture, and objects you love, the energy will naturally be elevated and support you in a positive way. Every time you see those items, you will feel good, relaxed, and vibrant. This is such an important point in feng shui because your environment is an extension of yourself, your inner self to be exact. During my consultations, I always point out the significance of decorating with objects that have deep meaning for my client. If there is any object they feel uncomfortable with, I recommend they remove it from the space because in essence they are telling the universe there is something they do not like about themselves.

Any object previously owned by another person will carry the energetic vibration of that person. If you know the individual who owned the object and you admired them, then that is the energetic vibration that you will experience from that object. On the other hand, if this individual was ill, mean-spirited, or mistreated you in any way, then those vibrational patterns will be imprinted within your space. This is why it is so important to rid yourself of possessions that have a negative association to them. Many times, however, people simply do not know the person who was the original owner of the object. This type of scenario is most common with estate sale buying. The best way to counteract any potential problematic energetic vibration is to consecrate the item through space clearing.

Why Space Clearing Can Maintain Healthy Living

Everything has energy. This is very profound and impacts your life on many levels. It means you have the ability to experience the objects within your environment in either a positive or negative way. It also means you have the opportunity to change that energy into anything you may desire in life.

An interesting concept followed by the Balinese people is called Sekala (the seen world) and Niskala (the unseen world). The Balinese understand that everything in the physical world is the result of its counterpart in the unseen world. Essentially, this suggests we can transform energy into our own reality and in the process manifest our desires. In order to do this some type of a catalyst is necessary.

The primary catalyst for the Balinese people is their ability to integrate their material world with their spiritual one. Here in the West, we tend to separate the two and, as a result, life can be more difficult and joyless. Like the Balinese people, we can also integrate both worlds in order to manifest all things in our life. The connection between the spirit and the material world should be one and not separate. The common denominator in these concepts is living in tune with nature, or God's world. Living close to the land puts us in sync with the universe allowing all else to naturally fall into place. When we disconnect ourselves from the earth, it causes a domino effect separating ourselves from our surroundings and each other. Feng shui provides that direct connection to nature and the ability to feel the energy within our surroundings.

Space clearing and consecration ceremonies are a wonderful catalyst to begin the transformation process. It can increase the energy level within a space and as a result directly impact your own energy level. This process of transmuting energy can assist you during difficult times like illness, divorce, separation, death, arguments, financial hardships, or any reoccurring problem. It can also aid in your health physically, mentally, and spiritually, improve intimacy and communication, change the atmosphere to feel better, assist you in manifesting what you want in life, improve finances, balance negative predecessor energy, and assist you during transitional periods, or times when you decide to move from one space to another.

<u>Basic Space Clearing Preparation & Procedures</u>

There are a number of space clearing techniques that can be utilized to transmute energy within a space. I personally use a combination of techniques based on the client's needs.

Consecrating Your Space

The key is to be comfortable with the ceremonial procedure and to adequately prepare yourself for the process. Below is one variation of a space clearing procedure I use that you can implement with great success.

1. Before taking on a space clearing session it is important you feel well rested, refreshed, healthy, and focused on your intentions.
2. If you share the space with other people it is important to inform them of what you are doing and offer them to take part in the ceremony.
3. Physically write down the reasons for the space clearing session and what you plan to achieve from it. The more specific you are about your intentions the greater the results will be.
4. Begin the process by giving your home a thorough cleaning. Remove all clutter, sweep, vacuum and mop all floors, wash windows and dust. Physical grime and clutter causes stuck energy and as a result the space clearing session will not be effective.
5. Avoid any potential distractions by disconnecting the phone, turning off the computer, stereo, television, or anything else that may disrupt your concentration.
6. Make sure you are well hydrated prior to the space clearing session. Try not to drink or eat during the process, as this will shift your personal energy flow and focus from the energy work you are trying to do.
7. Remove all jewelry or metal accessories from your body. Metal impacts energy frequencies and you do not want any interference while adjusting the energy in your space.
8. Keep close contact points to the natural earth energies during the session, as this will augment your own senses and assist energy movement. Walking through the space bare foot is one of the best ways to achieve this.
9. Set up a table near the front entrance in a position that allows full view of the entire space. This puts your body in a command position so physiologically you remain in a relaxed state.
10. Place the following on the table: A Tibetan bell, or any bell you might have, incense with an incense tray, sage stick with matches,

flower seeds, bowl of pure water with a few drops of holy water or your favorite essential oil, written intentions, and three white tea-light candles.

11. Obtain three additional trays and place one in the following rooms: kitchen, bedroom, and home office. On these trays place flower seeds around the three tea-light candles, incense stick with holder, and a copy of your intentions.

12. Wash your hands with water that has been exposed to sunlight, moonlight or a quartz crystal, as these components will naturally energize the water and will purify your energy prior to starting the ceremony.

13. Try to begin the ceremony between 11:00am and 1:00pm. This is the high point of the sun when the energetic level of the atmosphere is greatest.

14. Ask permission to space clear the home. Speak to the home as if it were a person and let it know your intentions. You may also ask your own spirit guides to assist you during the process.

15. Stand in the center of your home and close your eyes while taking three deep (belly) breaths. This will relax your body so you are more receptive to the energy in the space.

16. Light the three tea-light candles (represents heaven, man & earth) and the incense stick (use holder to avoid fire hazard) on each tray throughout the house. During the lighting process, recite your intentions to the Universe. This will automatically begin the process of attracting those desires into your life.

17. Light the sage stick and begin to walk the perimeter of the home in a clockwise direction to follow ch'i flow movement. Let the herb waft throughout the space hitting the corners, window frames, door jams, and base moldings. If your home has several levels, including a basement, then begin at the front door and continue around until you come to the basement door. Proceed down the basement and then back up to the main floor. Proceed to the next level until you arrive back at the front door and exit the door with your back first to symbolically draw low energy from the structure. You want to work from the bottom up, as that is how the energy levels stack (low to high). This replicates

the energy levels of the human chakra system, from the root to the crown (low to high).

18. The next phase is to create sound vibration. Sound will disperse any remaining stagnant energy from the space. The areas to focus on are the corners and dark alcoves. Just as dust tends to accumulate in these areas, stagnant energy tends to build at these points. You may use a bell or simply clap your hands for this step. Clapping hands is certainly easiest and doesn't require any additional tool. Always begin the clapping or bell chiming at the lowest point in the corner and gradually work your way up the corner until your hands are above your head. Areas where the energy is really stuck the clap or bell sound will be muffled. Simply continue to clap or chime the bell until the sound is sharp. Once you are satisfied with the tones in all the corners and dark areas and have returned to your starting point, draw the number 8 in the air with your hand or the bell to signify eternity or an everlasting energy. Wash your hands only if you used the clapping modality to release the stagnant energy.

19. It is time to set the intentions for the space. Take the bowl of pure water that is infused with the holy water or essential oil of your choice. Starting at the front door, walk around the space in a clockwise direction while flicking the infused water into the air. During the process, focus on your intentions and visualize them as a part of your life. Continue this process throughout the entire space.

20. Stand in the center of each room and take a Qigong stance known as "Nourishing Three Treasures." Stand with your feet wider than shoulder width apart and begin a deep inhalation while bending forward at the waist. Reach down with your hands and scoop up the earth energy from the ground. Raise this energy upward along the center of the front of your body (arms are soft and rounded as if holding a ball) and bring to chest level. Begin your exhalation and extend your arms and hands straight out and together in front of you (chest height). You are now offering your intentions to the Universe. Inhale and open your arms wide at shoulder height. Next, exhale and push your palms out as if you were pushing against a wall to each side of you. Inhale and begin raising your hands up toward the sky (palms facing out). Begin your

exhalation and bend forward from your waist, arms extended in a rounded position in front of you. Scoop up the earth ch'i again and lift it up again along the front of your body. Push your palms up toward the heavens and lift up onto your toes. Begin the last exhalation, opening your arms out to your sides with palms facing down and allow your hands to gently flow down. This movement is very powerful and will stimulate ch'i flow internally (in your body) and in the home. By doing this you will infuse the home with a "fresh" energy.

21. Next, go outside and sprinkle sea salt along the perimeter of the entire house. The salt will cleanse the outer aura of the house and reflect the yang energy of the sun to boost the surrounding ch'i.

22. The ceremony can be completed now with a prayer of thanks.

23. Put out all candles and incense sticks, remove all items from the table and take the flower seeds that are imbued with your intentions and sprinkle them outside returning them to Mother Earth.

24. Cleanse yourself by taking an Epsom salt bath.

Generally, a space clearing of this magnitude should only need to be done twice a year unless some major trauma occurs within the home. For periodic maintenance, simply walk through your home and chime a bell or clap, especially in the corners, while burning three candles or three incense sticks. Spritzing with any essential oil daily will also help boost the energy level. This type of a ceremony can be utilized for any of the aforementioned issues, including leaving a dwelling and moving into a new one.

Creating A Sacred Room

From a feng shui perspective, the home is an extension of your body, your well-being, and your livelihood. Throughout this book, the emphasis always comes down to your immediate surroundings. With that in mind, it is important to go a step further and create a space within your environment that you can go to on a daily basis to renew your soul and spirit. A room in the northeastern sector of your home works very well, as the energy resonates to self-cultivation and spirituality. Decorate this space with seven key components to nurture the mind, body, and soul.

1. <u>Sacred Objects:</u> These objects can be religious icons, spiritual books or CD's, any thing that represents spirituality to you, or the dreams you are manifesting for this world. You can actually create a small alter in this space that should include the four natural Greek elements (earth, wind or air, fire and water). Examples of the earth element are a crystal, healthy plant, or fresh flowers since they actually come from the earth. The fragrance of incense, essential oils, or a feather represents the wind or air energy. Candles illuminating a light source represent the fire energy. And finally, a fresh bowl of water acts as a purifier for the soul and obviously will represent the water energy.

2. <u>Incense & Candles:</u> The scent generated from incense represents a spiritual offering. In many religions, incense is an integral part of the ceremony and elevates the energy level within the space. The candles represent the light or the soul's illumination.

3. <u>Natural Elements:</u> Incorporating nature's elements into this space will bring you closer to connecting with the awesome energy of the universe. Plants, rocks, and crystals are just a few examples of natural elements that will augment this connection.

4. <u>Water:</u> Water is a source of nurturing, healing, and spiritual purification. Incorporating a water source in this room in the form of a fountain can be very spiritual and uplifting. The sounds created by the water can be very powerful and should mimic the sounds of a babbling brook, or stream in nature.

5. <u>Life Force:</u> Life force energy reminds you of the never-ending energy source in the universe. Energy cannot die; it simply changes its form. Therefore, by incorporating life forces in this space it can connect you to the infinite energy within your soul. Life force can be anything from fish, fresh flowers, to a healthy plant.

6. <u>Color:</u> Color is one of the most powerful elements within a space that can elevate the energy level and heal the mind, body and soul. It is thought that our soul emits a bright white light that is integrated throughout our physical body in our chakra system creating other color vibrations. Adding touches of purple to this sacred space will resonate to the seventh chakra, our

highest energy level, or spiritual realm. In traditional Buddhist monasteries, the colors red, yellow, blue, green, white and black are also used to support and sustain the spirituality of your life.

7. <u>Sacred Shapes of Geometry:</u> Geometric shapes represent the stages of "Becoming." It allows a direct access to the spiritual and material forces of creation. The ancients believed that by incorporating symbols of sacred geometry into the architecture would allow the soul to grow. These ancient earth designers constructed sacred patterns into their temples, monuments, and other structures in honor of their spiritual essence.

In order to fully understand the dynamics behind sacred geometry, one must realize the world is a natural phenomenon that is comprised of geometric forms. For example, this can be seen in our bodies as the double helix of DNA, in the structure of the cornea in the eye, and every other part of the body that follows this same predictable pattern. In the environment, it can be seen in the reoccurring shapes and fractals of leaves, flowers, seeds, the pattern of honeybees and other insects that live structured lives, the crystalline form of gems and stones, the swirl of a nautilus shell, the movement of the tides, the solar system, and the cycles of the moon. Sacred geometry is replicated in the vibrations of music (notes), the grid patterns seen on earth (ley lines), and in religious symbols, especially in Judaism, Christianity, and Hinduism.

These geometric forms have been a constant source of inspiration to scientists, philosophers, artists, musicians, and architects around the world. The perfect harmony displayed in these geometric forms always equals a measurement of (1.6180339887) and therefore was given the term of "The Golden Mean" or "Golden Ratio." This led Sir James Jeans, a British scientist during the mid 1800's, to pose the famous question: "Is God a mathematician?"

The ancient Greeks were also very interested in the Golden Ratio; as a result, it is seen in many works of art and architecture including the famous pyramids. The famous Fibonacci sequence (1,1,2,3,5,8,13,21,34, 55,...), where the generation of numbers occurs by adding the previous two numbers in the list together to form the next number, produces the Golden Ratio if you divide any number in the sequence by the one before it (55/34) = 1.61803. This configuration represents the search for absolute truth, love, or God.

Buildings or rooms that incorporate the Golden Mean principle and geometric form have a profound affect on your health and your psychic and spiritual state of being. Many earth designers who incorporate these principles into their architecture have also found the numbers one through six were manifested in the geometric design. The power of these numbers is believed to correspond to the cycles of creation. In the first chapter of the Bible (Genesis), it states that God created the earth in six days and on the seventh day he rested. Understand that the word "day" represents a cycle of approximately 24,000 years. This is the same time it takes our galaxy to rotate through 360 degrees or the 12 zodiac houses of Western Astrology. One cycle is equivalent to 2,000 years. That is the time it takes the galaxy to move through one house or sign. Hence, 12 signs or houses multiplied by 2,000 years gives us 24,000 years for one complete revolution. We have recently left the Piscean age (period when Christ was born) and have now entered the 6th cycle, or Age of Aquarius. If we observe these numbers, one through six, from a symbolic perspective we note the following:

- The Taoist philosophy of "One Begets Two" is based on the geometric shape of the circle. The circle is traditionally seen as God or one. Prior to the universe being created nothing existed but God. The diameter of the circle is its dynamic creation and symbolically represents the hidden nature of duality, thus the number two becomes the fundamental concept of creation.

- The number three is the power behind creation. Three defines the triad, or equilateral triangle. The triad or trinity represents the mind, body, and soul on a mortal level. In Christianity, it represents the Father, Son, and Holy Spirit. In Hinduism, it represents Brahma, Shiva, and Vishnu. In feng shui, it represents heaven, man, and earth. For man, this number allows the mind to focus so the body is able to do amazing things. A strong physical body expands your confidence and ability to obtain your higher goals in life. Knowledge increases and wisdom follows, so the spirit is able to reach a higher level. This sparks your intuitive nature that in turn expands the triad or trinity outward.

- The number four represents the creation in matter. It symbolizes the square, the four corners of the earth, and the cardinal points (E, S, W N). The use of this shape, along with a rectangle, represents a focus on the material world and unrealized potential in life. The square also creates the spiral through the relationship between the sides and the diagonal. The spiral of course is seen in the human DNA helix, seashells, pinecones, and configurations in seeds of sunflowers.

- o <u>The number five is the potential of all matter.</u> The five points or pentagram expands consciousness through the Golden Mean proportion. This is seen in Leonardo Da Vinci's famous work "Vitruvian Man," that depicted a naked male figure in two superimposed positions with his arms and legs apart and simultaneously drawn in a circle and square. It depicts the proportions of man that follow the Golden Mean Ratio.
- o <u>The number six represents the power of spirit brought into matter.</u> It is the symmetry and balance of two equilateral triangles, or the six-pointed star. These two triangles represent the trinity replicating itself in the material world and therefore it challenges man to see his own divinity within. The two overlapping circles also symbolize the number six. This is seen in the intersecting points of the circles that become the corresponding star points. This symbol is also seen as the Vesica Piscis, the fish symbol, or Piscean Christ.

When these symbolic number principles are incorporated within building and room designs, it can have a profound effect. Since your dwelling is seen as an extension of yourself, by creating spaces that support your dynamic being can sharpen your senses, improve your physical body, and reconnect you to your divine nature. When you choose to build and design your enviroment with more synthetic materials rather than natural materials, you are disregarding nature in the process. Therefore, you shut down your true nature and, as a result, this can lead to disharmony, imbalance, and disease. There is an old Chinese proverb that says, "When there is order in the house, there is order in the nation, where there is order in the nation, there is peace in the world." Below are some ideas of how to incorporate sacred symbols and the Golden Mean Ratio into your space.

- o <u>Labyrinths:</u> A labyrinth is simply a system of paths that can be easy to get lost in. The design of a labyrinth eases the mind into

Consecrating Your Space

a meditative state. You can create a small labyrinth in your yard or garden by simply creating pathways with hedges, shrubs, stones, or mosaic tiles. You can also purchase a geometric pattern of a labyrinth and hang it on the wall of your sacred room, or area where you meditate. This geometric form activates the subconscious mind and symbolizes a winding path to the divine source.

o   Nautilus Shell: Keep a nautilus shell or ammonite fossil displayed in your home. The spiral shape conforms to the Golden Mean Ratio and exudes divine harmony.

o   Mandala: Mandala is Sanskrit for circle and symbolizes transformation, healing and unity with the creator. A mandala can be placed on a coffee table or shelf. You can purchase a sand tray mandala with a swinging pendulum. When the pendulum moves it will create a sacred design formation in the sand.

o   Plants: Living plants represent the geometric aspect in nature known as fractals. The way leaves grow around the stem and the veining of the leaf is a sacred principle that will keep you connected to nature.

o   Spiral Designs: Any spiral designs creating a swirling movement rotating downward to a center point, then upward, are extremely powerful sacred shapes. Many times Native American pottery depicts these designs.

o   Sacred Shapes: Incorporate seashells, crystals, ferns, leaves, circles, triangles, pyramids, cubes, and hexagons in your space.

o   Artwork: Incorporate art with landscape scenes, flowers, or spiral designs.

o   Kaleidoscope: Get a Kaleidoscope and add it to your room décor. Use it frequently and experience the sacred shapes created by the movement. The best ones to use are those that have the small color chips.

o   Golden Mean Ratio: You can incorporate the Golden Mean ratio in any room that is odd shaped. Simply measure the width of the room and then multiply it by the Golden Mean Ratio (1.618) to find the perfect length. For example, a room with a width of 14 feet multiplied by 1.618 equals 22.652 or 23 feet. This is the perfect length for a room that is 14 feet wide. Simply design the furniture around these dimensions and create a separate area for any additional odd space. This works especially well when a room is long and narrow. You may also use this same concept in an odd shape yard. You can delineate the divine proportion area from another area by planting a natural barrier with hedges or shrubbery.

The human body resonates to nature on a cellular and conscious level. By designing your enviroment with nature's symbols and geometric forms found in those symbols, you then can create a space that nurtures you instead of one that drains you. This type of architecture and interior design supports the principles of universal harmony and nurtures your own senses and creativity in life.

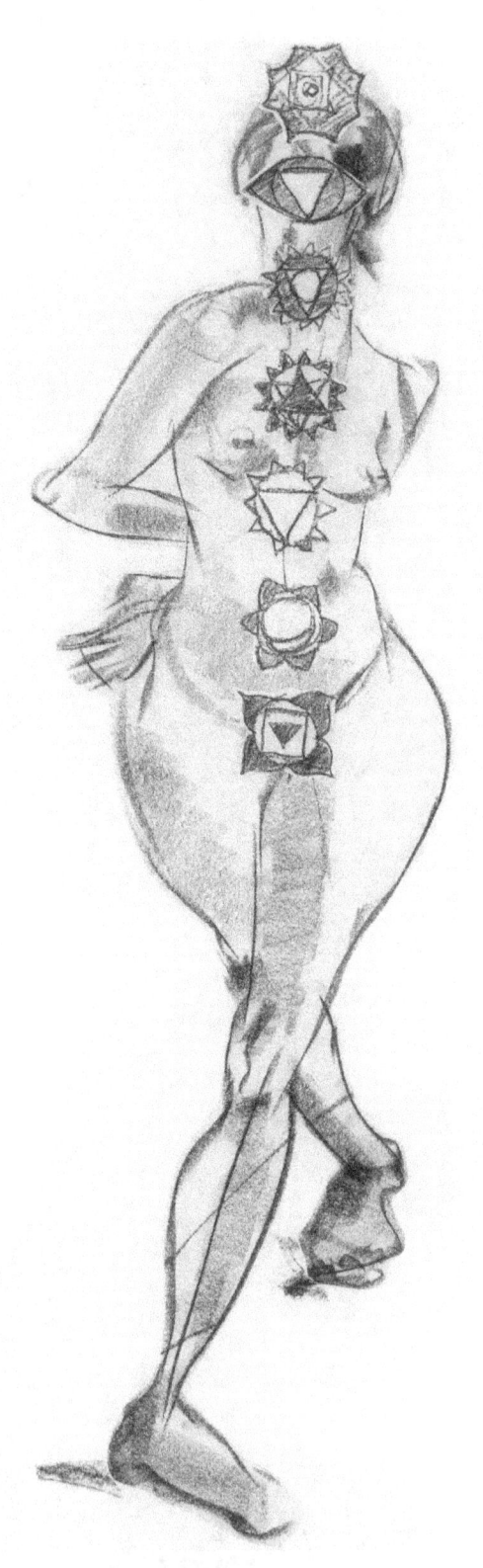

9
Aligning The Mind, Body & Soul

"Meditation is the tongue of the soul and the language of our spirit."

Jeremy Taylor

According to the Taoist viewpoint, all energy within the universe is a result of the interaction between yin and yang. The result of the interplay between these two interdependent polarities establishes three realms of energy within the universe. These three types of energy are known as cosmic energy, universal energy, and earth energy. The cosmic ch'i is how the Taoist philosopher believes the planets, stars, human cells, and all other life forms are nourished. Universal ch'i energy is a result of radiating forces of all the galaxies, stars, and planets. Earth ch'i encompasses all energies of Mother Earth and is activated by the electromagnetic field created by the earth's rotation.

In Taoist practice, human energy is believed to be the highest manifestation of cosmic light and the intermediary between heaven and earth forces. It is believed the human body has three energy centers located on the vertical axis of the body. These three centers are called Tan Tiens and are positioned from low to high (pelvic, torso, head) and believed to act as energy points for the physical body, soul, and spirit. These three Tan Tiens represent the three main stages of spirituality in Taoism. The lower Tan Tien (pelvic to belly region) corresponds directly to the physical body. A strong lower Tan Tien facilitates a healthy body and abundant life force. This level naturally progresses to the middle Tan Tien located at the solar plexus to heart region. This middle Tan Tien is said to correspond to the soul. Here is where we develop unconditional love, morals, and virtue. When this level is strong we develop an intimate connection with mankind and, as a result, we begin to nourish our spiritual self. The spiritual self is the third and upper

Tan Tien and is located in the head region. When this Tan Tien level is developed, we experience spiritual enlightenment and begin to share the "light" with others. Taoist teachings such as Qigong (pronounced "chee gung") and Tai-Chi work with exercises and meditations to cultivate and strengthen the inner ch'i building these Tan Tiens points.

There are hundreds of methods of Qigong, combining teachings of Buddhist, Taoist, and Confucian methods. Today, the Chinese have adapted these different teachings into a multi-discipline format. The overall premise is to train the body to absorb vital ch'i. Many people in the Far East practice this moving meditation outdoors so they are in contact with Mother Earth.

There are generally fifteen precursor principles to learning disciplines like Tai-Chi and Qigong to assist with a healthier life style. Below is a list of the basic principles behind Tai-Chi and Qigong practice. It is recommended to train with an experienced practitioner in these disciplines. Many times your local community college or park system offers such programs.

Tai-Chi & Qigong Basic Principles

Principle 1: "Let Go!" This principle is all about releasing any emotional, physical or mental blockages. By focusing on the lower Tan Tien (belly area), it will help to release these constraints.

Principle 2: "Experience Yin And Yang Polarity Within Yourself." There are specific Qigong and Tai-Chi movements that the body goes through to distribute tension evenly. By understanding the yin (negative) and yang (positive) qualities, creative possibilities flow into your life.

Principle 3: "Listen To Your Heart Beats And Breathing." In order to improve ch'i within your body, you need to make a connection between your heart beating and your breathing. Taoist teachers express this principle as Wu-Chi, meaning feeling alone and full at the same time. All judgment qualities must be released.

Principle 4: "Coordinate Movement From The Tan Tien (Belly Region)." Consistent and smooth body movements take a cyclic pattern mimicking the ebb and flow in nature. This action relieves tension while improving ch'i flow.

Principle 5: "Meditate on Stillness in Motion." Tai-Chi and Qigong focus on energy from the feet upwards through the meridian channels (pathways of energy flow). With practice, this energy flow promotes peace and abundance.

Principle 6: "Be Effortless. Flow With Life And Life Flows With You." The body moves smoothly with these exercise movements. Trust in inner knowing and harmonious solutions will prevail.

Principle 7: "Enjoy The Art of Being And Feel Grateful For Every Little Step of Progress You Make." Be grateful for all your accomplishments no matter how large or small. When we show gratitude, it encourages ch'i flow and improves all of the body systems.

Principle 8: "Become A Fountain of Smiling Ch'i." This is sometimes referred to as our "Inner Smile Bright." Smiling to our internal organs and appreciating all they do reinforces healthy immune systems. Well-trained practitioners can go beyond focusing on limb movement and connect to the inner organs.

Principle 9: "Transform Stress And Conserve Ch'i Energy In Your Internal Organ." Qigong exercises allow you to draw on the three ch'i levels (earth, human, and heavenly) and transform stress into health.

Principle 10: "Use Ch'i Energy To Uplift And Use Spiritual Movement To Ground Yourself." This principle teaches the body to become fluid in movement, which is essential for proper ch'i movement. Ch'i energy naturally ascends and then descends requiring fluid bodily movements.

Principle 11: "Use Ch'i To Purify And Transport Vitality To Any Part of The Body That Needs It." Since the human body is comprised of more than seventy percent water, it has a natural affinity to create fluid movement. This is the way ch'i modulates within the body and therefore can be projected to any desired area.

Principles 12-15: "The Four Seasons Rhythms." According to Traditional Chinese Medicine, the heart governs the ch'i in the body pumping blood in four distinct phases. These phases are said to mimic the four seasons in nature. For example, Spring represents all new cells. Summer is the expansion or growth of these cells. Autumn represents the distribution of nutrients throughout the body; And Winter is when the cells contract. These same movements are seen in Tai-Chi and Qigong exercises resulting in balance and harmony in life.

The aforementioned are the basic principles behind Tai-Chi and Qigong exercises. By practicing these moving meditations you can reinforce proper ch'i flow within the body resulting in a more centered approach to physical, mental, and spiritual health.

The Human Aura

The human aura is encapsulated by an electromagnetic field from the top of your head to your feet. The electrical component relates to your conscious mind and processes of the central nervous system. The magnetic component corresponds to your subconscious mind, your emotions, and autonomic nervous system (those areas we do not have control over) such as breathing. This energy field is in a constant state of flux and varies from person to person depending on your physical make-up.

The human aura extends to seven layers whereby the first three are most recognized and seen by others. These first three layers are positioned closest to the physical body. It consists of the Physical layer, Ethric layer, and Vital Auric layer.

Physical Layer: The Physical layer is situated closest to the physical body and is approximately four inches in depth. It takes on the shape of the human body and it is the most common layer seen by energy workers. It is the densest of all the layers and can experience the senses of sight, sound, smell, touch, and taste.

Ethric Layer: This layer also mimics the form of the physical body and is very pronounced in people who exercise frequently. This layer sits very close to the body, approximately two inches away. The main function for this layer is to establish a network system for the vibrational energy of the body organ systems. This is the layer that trained energy workers can evaluate for a potential illness. Dr. Richard Gerber comments in his book "Vibrational Medicine," "The ethric body is a holographic energy template that guides the growth and development of the physical body." From this comment, we can ascertain that the ethric body is a precursor to the health of the physical body.

Vital Auric Layer: This layer directly corresponds to your energy levels. Generally, if you are energetic, this layer is very healthy and well aligned. If, on the other hand, this layer is weak, then you will feel lethargic and depleted of energy.

Aligning The Mind, Body & Soul

There are four outer layers of the auric system that are very difficult to see unless you are a trained energy worker. The four outer layers consist of the Emotional Aura, Lower Mental Aura, Upper Mental Aura, and Spiritual Aura.

<u>Emotional Aura:</u> This layer will also follow the shape of the physical body and contain many different color hues depending on the emotions of the individual. It is approximately a hand width away from the body and reflects your emotions, how you interact with others energetically, and how you use your emotions when making decisions.

<u>Lower Mental Aura:</u> This layer reflects your daily activities and thought processes. It is your daily routine in life. Most of the time this is the aura level you remain stuck in throughout life.

<u>Upper Mental Aura:</u> This layer corresponds to your higher intellect or inner wisdom. This is your intuitive knowledge that connects you to your soul's purpose. It generally appears as a yellow light and extends between three to eight inches from the entire body. This is a layer that many of us fail to explore and develop. As a result, you remain stuck in the lower mental aura.

<u>Spiritual Aura:</u> This is the most outer layer and is approximately an arms length away from the body. It contains all the information about your life experiences and is responsible for shaping your soul's purpose for this lifetime. This is your connection to the divine. It is the layer that connects you to the Universe, or the first Taoist principle that states: "All is one."

Exercise To Develop A Healthy Aura

One of the easiest ways to begin to develop a sense of your aura is to stroke your body slowly without touching it. Simply hold your hands approximately eight inches from the top of your head and slowly move them downward outlining your body shape. Close your eyes during this exercise and tune into the stroking motion. You will begin to feel energy in the form of heat, coolness, or perhaps slight pressure. This is your body's electromagnetic field, or aura.

At times the auric layers can become weak due to illness, injury or our environmental surroundings. Spaces that contain high EMF's, synthetics, fluorescent lighting, and high positive ions can impact the health and vibrancy of the auric field. You can pretty much control all of these factors through proper diet, exercise, resolving any emotional constraints, and following good feng shui practice. Once you have these areas under control, then you can maintain the auric field through cleansing and visualization.

Cleansing & Visualization

Begin by placing your hands approximately eight inches from your body and wiping the aura on one side of your body from the top of your head downward outlining the shape of your body. Before proceeding to the other side, shake your hands to remove any stagnant energy. To make a bigger impact on the cleansing procedure, set an intention that you are washing your auric field. Once you have completed this step, you are ready to begin the visualization process.

The visualization process requires a meditative state. Find a relaxed position where you will not be disturbed. Make sure the environment is comfortable and the temperature is on the warmer side. Begin with deep breathing (belly breaths) to relax your mind and body. Visualize a pure white light entering your body from the top of your head and slowly filling every area of your body. Visualize inhaling this white light so it circulates throughout your lungs and circulatory system. This mental exercise symbolizes a cleansing of any stagnant areas. Exhale the stagnant energy while inhaling the healing white light. Visualize this white light emanating from your body and vibrating outward. End the meditation by drawing the white light inward, so it encapsulates your body at the spiritual auric layer (arms length from the body). Try to perform this visual meditation on a daily basis to cleanse your aura.

The Colorful Auric System

The human body extends beyond its physical state carrying energy fields with dynamic color hues. These colors, encapsulated within the auric layers, are in a constant state of movement and change in color depending upon your life experiences and emotional make-up. Some people can see auras and interpret the meanings behind the color matrix. More technical approaches to reading the auric layers are captured through Kirlian photography or Polycontrast Interference Photography (PIP). These forms of photography are able to capture the different light forms that surround the human body. These pictures are then analyzed and can determine the well-being of a person.

Meaning Of Auric Colors

Scientifically, color is a sensation produced by the brain by light that is transmitted from an object to the eye activating different cones in the retina. The body seems to react to color inducing different emotions and behavior. When different colors are seen in the auric system, it can determine what an individual is experiencing. Below is a list of some basic auric colors and their meanings.

<u>Red:</u> When the color red is seen in the aura, it generally means a person is experiencing powerful emotions such as anger, rage or passion. Since red is a very energetic color, it may also mean the person is very active in their life.

<u>Orange:</u> In color theory, orange is a color that represents joy and creativity. When this color is seen in the aura, it usually means the individual is involved with creative activities, very social, or experiencing a significant change in their life.

<u>Yellow:</u> This is the color of intellect and thought processes. People who have a lot of yellow in their aura are education oriented and very cerebral in nature.

<u>Green:</u> Green is a calming color and reinforces balance and harmony. This is a wonderful color in the human aura and many times is indicative of a healing process. However, an overabundance of green may indicate the individual is jealous of another person.

<u>Blues/Indigo:</u> Blues are very healing in nature and can indicate a person who uses their energy to heal others. A predominance of indigo corresponds directly to the third eye chakra and our intuitive capabilities.

<u>Purple:</u> This color resonates to the seventh chakra. An aura highly concentrated with this color indicates a person who is spiritually motivated in life.

<u>Black:</u> A great deal of black in the aura is indicative of a person who is depressed, seriously ill, or misusing drugs. Since the body is being compromised, the otherwise vibrate colors associated with a healthy mind, body, and soul is not seen.

<u>White:</u> The color white always represents purity, freshness, truth and wisdom. These characteristics are difficult to fully achieve in life; therefore, a pure white aura is rare to come by.

The aforementioned colors are just a few examples found in the human auric system. There are various other color combinations that can be found in the human aura and can change depending on the experiences encountered by the individual.

The Human Chakra System

Just as the auric system represents energetic layers of the human body, the chakras and nadis represent vibrational energy centers and channels respectively. The term chakra literally means, "wheel" in Sanskrit because the human chakras are wheel-like depressions that exist on the surface of the ethric auric layer. Nadis in Sanskrit means "pipe or vein." These nadis are an intricate network of channels carrying the vital life force ch'i or prana into the fourteen main channels or meridians that connect to the chakra system.

The chakra system is actually quite complex and believed to contain some eighty-eight thousand points in the human body. However, most of the energy transference occurs within seven main chakra points. Six of these main chakras align with the vertical axis of the spine, while the seventh opens at the top of the head. Each chakra rotates pulling energy inward and then pulsating it back out. The disc-like shape of each chakra looks like the lotus flower and extends approximately four inches in all directions. Some schools of thought believe the chakras rotate in a clockwise direction, while others believe the chakras will alternate directional spin (clockwise and counterclockwise) based on the individual's gender. For example, if the root chakra is rotating counterclockwise for a man, then the root chakra for the female will rotate clockwise. The basic premise is balance and harmony (yin and yang) between a man and a woman.

The Seven Major Chakras

The seven major chakras (root, sacral, solar plexus, heart, throat, third-eye and crown) contain four energy channels and correspond to specific body systems and life situations. The first energy channel spirals upward from the root (pelvic) chakra to the crown (head) chakra. The second energy channel spirals downward towards the root or base chakra creating a grounding energy with the earth. The third channel projects outward from the front of the body, while the forth energy channel projects outward from the back of the body. These four energy channels are responsible for absorbing "Universal Source Energy" and transferring it to the human body for healing purposes. Below is a list of the seven main chakras with their corresponding body systems and life associations.

Chakra Energy Descriptions

1. **Root Chakra:** The first chakra is known as the root or base chakra. It is located at the pelvic or genital region of the physical body. The spin rotation is the slowest of all the chakras and the energy vortex opens downward. In Sanskrit, this chakra is referred to as Muladhara and is associated with the color red. This chakra corresponds to the spinal column, kidneys, and adrenal system. The primary energy associated with this chakra is survival. On an intrinsic level it is how you take care of your basic needs in life such as food and shelter. By and large, you are able to take care of these necessities; however, you can deplete this energy when you disconnect yourself from nature.

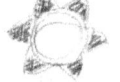

2. **Sacral Chakra:** This chakra is referred to as the belly chakra and is located at the lower abdominal area. The spin rotation is slightly faster than the root chakra and is associated with the color orange. In Sanskrit, this chakra is known as Svadhisthana. Its energy vortex opens to the front and relates to the reproductive system, specifically the testes and ovaries. The primary energy associated with this chakra is creativity and pleasure in life. This can include procreation, sexuality, and the passions you have in life.

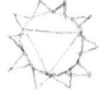

3. **Solar Plexus Chakra:** This chakra is located slightly above the naval region. The spin rotation accelerates at this point and the vortex opens towards the front of the body. In Sanskrit this chakra is known as Manipura. It is associated with the yellow color of the sun and corresponds to

the gall bladder, liver, and pancreas. The primary energy associated with this chakra is self-confidence. It is all about your ability to rely on your personal power and self-esteem.

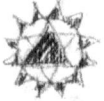
4. <u>Heart Chakra:</u> This chakra is located at heart level. It is the center of the entire chakra system connecting the three lower chakras to the three upper chakras. The spin rotation continues to escalate rising continuously as you move up the spinal column. The color association for this chakra is green. In Sanskrit this chakra is known as Anahata. It corresponds to the heart, blood vessels, circulatory system, vagus nerve, and thymus. The primary energy is one of unconditional love. This is your ability to love without conditions. It is the ability to connect with the Universal Source Energy, or God.

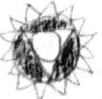
5. <u>Throat Chakra:</u> This chakra is located behind the Adam's Apple. The spin rotation is very fast and the energy vortex opens towards the front and back. It is associated with the blue color of the sky and is known as Vissuddha in Sanskrit. This chakra corresponds to the lungs, larynx, and thyroid. Its primary energy associated with this chakra center is communication. This includes verbal, body, and telepathic forms of communication.

6. <u>Third-Eye Chakra:</u> This chakra is located between the eyebrows. There is an extremely fast rotational spin, where the energy vortex opens outward. It is associated with the color indigo and referred to as Ajna in Sanskrit. It corresponds to the ears, nose, lower brain, nervous system, and left eye. The primary energy association is your higher mental powers. It is about your intuition, psychic abilities, and precognition. This chakra is about using your mind for a positive impact on your life.

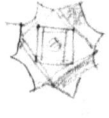
7. <u>Crown Chakra:</u> This chakra is sometimes referred to as the spiritual chakra. It is located in the pineal gland, or at the top of the head. The energy vortex opens upward and its rotational spin is faster than the previous six chakras. It is associated with the color purple and referred to as Sahsrara in Sanskrit. The primary energy source for this

chakra is inner knowing or enlightenment. This is the chakra that directly connects us to the divine source of the universe (God). When this chakra is fully developed, enlightenment, or the highest level of consciousness is achieved.

These are the seven main chakras whereby six of them align the spinal column and the seventh opens to the top of the head. Every chakra rotates perpetually and is in a constant receptive mode to the environment and Universal Energy Source. The spin rotation and energy vortex depends on how healthy and consciously developed a person is. Any illness and lack of spiritual development can produce a sluggish motion in the chakras. Depending on the type of illness and the affected body system, the corresponding chakra can decelerate in rotation in comparison to the other chakras.

Aligning The Chakras

The chakras are susceptible to your external and internal environment. If you recall in chapters five and six, every part of the dwelling is associated with a body system. Since each chakra is also associated with a body system, it behooves you to inspect your home for anything in disrepair. This is one way to support the physical body. Obviously, a balanced diet, regular exercise, meditation, and prayer are additional dynamics that can impact the chakra system. Below are some examples of how to align the chakras.

Crystals: Crystals are natural elements that are derived from Mother Earth. For thousands of years they have been used to heal, protect, and adorn the body. Many cultures throughout the world incorporated crystals as a treatment modality for body ailments.

Today, crystals are being used in a similar manner. Their natural ability to transmit, transform, repel, and attract energy, make them wonderful accoutrements to feng shui practice and healing measures.

Crystals work especially well in protecting the auric and chakra systems. Their energetic vibration can align, cleanse, activate, and calm these subtle systems. When using crystals to align the chakras, it is important to place the crystal either to the front or back of the chakra so direct contact is made for alignment and healing to occur.

Basic Crystal Alignment Procedures

- Choose the appropriate crystal for each chakra (see chart below)
- Make sure the crystal is cleared (see Cleansing Crystals on page 185)
- Set a healing intention on the crystal by cupping it in your hands and reciting a positive affirmation
- Repeat the intention process for each chakra
- Wear comfortable clothing
- Choose a space where you will not be interrupted
- Lie on your back and place the appropriate crystal on each chakra point
- Close your eyes and visualize each chakra wheel spinning and projecting the associated color outward (ie: root chakra is the color red)
- Remove crystals and cleanse them
- Store crystals in a silk pouch

Chakras	Aura
Crown: Selenite, Kunzite, Celestite	Protector: Amber
Third-Eye: Sodalite, Garnet, Fluorite	Cleanses: Amethyst
Throat: Turquoise, Amethyst, Kunzite	Aligns: Citrine
Heart: Rose Quartz, Adventurine, Rhodonite	Psychic Protector: Fluorite
Solar Plexus: Tiger's Eye, Citrine, Malachite	Healing: Green Tourmaline
Sacral: Topaz, Blue Jasper, Citrine, Carnelian	Protects Energy: Labradorite
Root: Bloodstone, Obsidian, Red Jasper	Strengthens & Grounds: Magnetite & Smokey Quartz

*Keep stones for aura balancing on your body

Fig. 35

Aligning The Mind, Body & Soul

Quartz Crystal Chakra Alignment

You can align the chakras daily in fifteen minutes using small terminating quartz crystal points. You will need eight crystal points for this chakra alignment procedure.

- Cleanse crystal points
- Wear comfortable clothing
- Choose a space where you will not be interrupted
- Lie on your back in a relaxed position (Shavasana- dead man's pose in yoga practice)
- Place two terminating crystal points on each thigh with the crystal point directed upward toward your head
- Take two more crystal points and place them on your chest (heart chakra) pointed upward
- Place two crystal points on the third-eye chakra (brow) with the pointed side directed downward
- Place the last two crystal points in the palm of each hand with the points directed upward
- Lay in this position for fifteen minutes visualizing each chakra spinning with the appropriate color vibrating outward

Cleansing Crystals

Since crystals can absorb energy and emit energy, it is important they are cleansed periodically. There are a number of ways to purify a crystal and any of the following modalities are fine to use.

<u>Sunlight/Moonlight:</u> Placing your crystals in direct sunlight or moonlight for several hours will naturally cleanse crystals. Any crystal that is yellow, orange or red has a natural affinity to the sun, while those that are white, clear, or gray gravitate towards the moon's energy.

<u>Incense or Herbs:</u> Burning incense or herbs will create an energetic smoke that will cleanse the crystal. Let the smoke waft completely around the crystal to purify its energy.

<u>Essential Oils:</u> Spraying your crystals with any essential oil will instantly clear and refresh them. Choose a scent that feels uplifting and refreshing when using this cleansing modality.

<u>Rain/Running Water/Salt Water:</u> Using water to purify your crystals is one of the most energetic ways to cleanse a crystal. Whether you hold them under running water from a faucet, leave them out in a rain storm, submerge them in a stream, or place them in a bowl with dissolved sea salt, these are all excellent ways to naturally cleanse them. To further energize the crystal, allow them to dry in direct sunlight.

Healing The Chakras With Color & Sound

We know that imbalances in the chakras can be the result of your environment, diet, and activity levels. The chakras can also be affected by unreleased emotions, traumatic experiences, or just a lack of being nurtured with love. These imbalances create energy blockages causing the chakras to spin irregularly and become distorted. This can trigger physical affects including feelings of lethargy or general malaise.

The chakras can be treated with color meditations and sound vibrations to rebalance their spin rotation and projection field. If the energy is deficient in a particular chakra, then incorporating that color in your décor, clothing, jewelry, stones or visualization can strengthen that chakra. On the other hand, if the chakra has excessive energy, then incorporating the "antidote" color (opposite color of chakra) into your surroundings, clothing, or through visualization can rebalance the chakra.

In order to determine if a chakra is sluggish or has excessive energy, pay attention to the behavioral qualities associated with each chakra and determine if there is a shift in either direction. When determining the antidote color, simply refer to a color wheel chart and locate the color that is opposite of that chakra color.

Basic Color Meditation

1. Wear comfortable clothing.
2. Choose a quiet room where you will not be disturbed.
3. Sit upright with a straight spine.
4. Close your eyes and visualize each chakra from the root to the crown.
5. Breathe deeply into each chakra beginning with the root chakra while visualizing the associated color filling that chakra. Then visualize that same color throughout your entire body, and finally

into the entire space you are in.
6. Proceed through each chakra in the same format until your reach the seventh or crown chakra.
7. Once you complete the color meditation, begin to visualize a clear passageway of free flowing energy from the root chakra to the crown chakra. This final meditation step will ground the chakras and create a big difference in your life.

Rebalancing The Chakras With Sound

Sound therapy is a combination of ancient and modern day knowledge that has been used for therapeutic purposes for thousands of years. Since sound is a result of vibrational waves, it becomes a perfect modality to tune the chakras. How is this possible? Each chakra vibrates to a tonal quality found in musical notes and vowel sounds.

When sounds are created by either vocals or an instrument, the vibrational energy of each chakra returns to its original healthy state. The following chart lists the corresponding musical notes, vowels sounds, and mantras for each chakra that can be used for a sound tuning meditation.

Chakra	Note	Vowel	Mantra
Base	C	u (ooh)	LAM
Sacral	D	o (low)	VAM
Solar Plexus	E	o (God)	RAM
Heart	F	ah	YAM
Throat	G	eh	HAM
Third-Eye	A	e (ee)	KSHAM
Crown	B	m	OM

Fig. 36

Balancing The Chakras With Essential Oils

The use of essential oils dates back to 7000 BC, when the Egyptians used blends of fragrant oils for mummification. The Greeks and Romans were also responsible for using aromatic plants to adorn their bodies during special events and to anoint their temples. The Bible also makes mention of essential oils like Spikenard, Frankincense, and Myrrh. The point being made here is essential oils have a long history for therapeutic usage, even though today many think it is a new concept.

The reason why essential oils are such a powerful source of therapy is two-fold. First, they carry an electromagnetic charge from the original plant source, so the full benefit of the flower essence is used. Second, the olfactory process in the human body reacts to these scents by activating the limbic system of the brain. This brain structure is very old and is referred to as the "emotional brain." When this area of the brain is activated a physiological response occurs, releasing neurotransmitters such as serotonin and endorphins. Serotonin helps the body to relax while endorphins give the body a natural high.

Since there is a vibrational energy directly connected to essential oils via the electromagnetic charge from the plant, this makes them a wonderful tool for cleansing and balancing the chakras. Below is a chart of the seven chakras and their corresponding essential oils.

Chakra	Oils
Base	Sandalwood, Patchouly, Ylang Ylang
Sacral	Sandalwood, Patchouly, Sage, Ylang Ylang
Solar Plexus	Fennel, Juniper
Heart	Bergamot, Rose, Peppermint, Cinnamon
Throat	Sandalwood, Rose, Eucalyptus
Third-Eye	Frankincense, Cedarwood, Mandarin
Crown	Jasmine, Frankincense, Elemi

Fig. 37

Meditation

Meditation is a highly complex activity that can achieve harmony within. The basic premise is to purify the mind by clearing all mental images and thoughts. One of the most common meditation practices is yoga, more specifically, "Bhaki" yoga. This type of yoga focuses the mind on the Divine. It is a very common form of quiet meditation that is practiced in many religions including Buddhism, Christianity, and Judaism.

The benefits of this quiet contemplation on a daily basis are endless. It combats daily life stresses, leaves you feeling refreshed, triggers endorphins (nature's natural opiates), boosts the immune system, and gives you an overall sense of calm.

There are many different meditation techniques that you can engage in. The key is to find one that resonates with you comfortably so you are able to practice it for twenty minutes a day. Below is one example of how you can prepare your mind for meditation practice.

Basic Steps For Meditating

Step 1:
- Wash your hands and face to refresh and cleanse your body
- Wear comfortable clothing and remove your shoes
- Choose a quiet comfortable space where you will not be disturbed

Step 2:
- Sit or lie in a comfortable position
- Close your eyes
- Lay your hands with palms open either on your lap (sitting) or along side your body (shavasana-dead man's pose in yoga)

Step 3:
- Breath in harmony with the universal ch'i force by inhaling through your nose allowing your belly to fully rise
- Take deep long breaths and absorb every thing good during the inhalation process

- Exhale through your nose so you feel your stomach contract towards your spine

- Release all bad thoughts during the exhalation process

- Slowly continue the breathing process

- Try to empty your mind of any thoughts or images by using a mantra (word or words) if necessary

- Continue this process for twenty minutes a day

The mind-body connection is the final and most powerful link to connecting with the Universal Energy Source. By preparing and sustaining your environment with the vibrations of nature, your innate ability to balance your inner self is awakened. This in turn aligns you to a higher vibration of your soul's intention. When you vibrate with your soul's intention, you attract all that is good into your life. This is the Universal Law of Attraction. Everything you desire in life is available to you based on these principles. You create your own resistance through your thoughts and behavior. By balancing your environment through feng shui applications you in turn align your physical, mental and spiritual essence. There is unlimited abundance to fill your life, if you let it in.

Epilogue

Chinese culture, as we know it today, is 5,000 years of societal transformation and development. Over numerous millennia, their diligence, precision, and observations enabled crucial discoveries of time, seasons, directions, and concepts of ch'i (energy), yin, yang, five elements, and the great philosophical book, the I Ching. These discoveries were the basis for the principles of Feng Shui.

Throughout the pages of this book, life force energy (ch'i) was examined thoroughly by the human body and the environment. You discovered how the quality of ch'i impacts your life experience through the land, building dynamics, interior design, activities, and diet.

After reading this book, you know how to recognize problematic building and land formations and how they can impact your mind and body. Throughout the pages you learned how to manage problematic designs by utilizing the principles covered in this book so you can create your desired life.

Refining your space was cultivated in chapter eight. In this section, you discovered the dynamics of space clearing, sacred geometric form, and how they can renew your home, body, and mind. These refining techniques are powerful in uniting yourself with your soul's intention.

The final link is the mind-body connection. Your innate ability to balance your internal ch'i (energy) through meditation and regulation of the subtle auric and chakra energy fields is the most powerful link to the universal energy source. This is the basis behind the law of attraction and the exclusive cipher to your aspirations.

Here's to a healthy life filled with high vitality and prosperity.

Peace & Many Blessings!

Mary Jane Kasliner

Appendix

Western Zodiac:

When most people think of Astrology they think: "What is my Horoscope?" Technically, the horoscope is an overview of the planetary positions at the moment of birth. The planets are actually the biggest component to an astrological chart. They are considered to be the "What" in astrology and are responsible for our motivations in life. The signs are simply "How" these planetary urges manifest in our behavior, whereas the houses, twelve to be exact, represent the "Where" component in astrology.

Notoriously, the houses fall into a fixed aspect of one's life such as self, personal security, mentality, personal roles, creativity, work, significant others, shared resources, ideology, social roles, social creativity, and self-denial. However, the reality is, no two people experience the same environmental conditions in life. Therefore, the houses of the horoscope are more or less concepts that will vary from one person to the next.

The astrological chart acts as a guide for the individual who can then apply their motivations in life (planets) and manifested behaviors (signs) according to their personal experiences (houses). With that being said, an astrological reading becomes a self-discovery process, whereby the individual is the pilot, and the astrologer is the co-pilot. Below are basic descriptions of the astrological signs only. These descriptions are a combination of how the planets react in a sign, along with the common characteristics of the sign. It is important to note that the sign descriptions are by no means the character of an individual who is born under a specific sign (sun sign). Astrological interpretations are very complicated and take into consideration many different components that comprise the whole. It is beyond the scope of this book to point out every dynamic that comes into play in the interpretive process.

<u>Aries - March 21 - April 20:</u> This is the first sign of the zodiac. It is classified as a cardinal mode and therefore has an initiatory type of energy. It is also the first of three fire signs, making this a very spirited and impulsive energy. Planets that are positioned in this sign have a natural driving force about them.

Aries is also known as the "Ram" and the sign of the pioneer and warrior leader. There is a sense of enthusiasm, risk-taking, and extrovert nature about this sign. However, Aries also has qualities of impatience, procrastination, selfishness, and aggressive behavior. This sign is most compatible with Gemini, Sagittarius, and Aquarius. Libra is the opposite sign in the zodiac.

<u>Taurus - April 21 - May20:</u> Taurus is the second sign of the zodiac. It is considered to be a stable or fixed mode, making this energy very grounded or stabilizing in nature. It is also an earth sign giving the energy a rather empirical or experiential way about it. Planets that are positioned in this sign function in a more practical or cautious nature; therefore, it is important for past experience to take the directive for this sign.

Taurus is referred to as the "Bull" and is the sign of the builder and the earth we stand on. Taurus is also a sign of great patience, determination, and reliability. The downside to Taurus is the possessive, inflexible, greedy and self-indulgent tendencies. This sign is most compatible with Capricorn, Pisces, Virgo, and Cancer. Scorpio is the opposite sign in the zodiac.

<u>Gemini - May 21 - June 21:</u> Gemini is the third sign of the zodiac. It is considered to be a flexible or adaptable mode, making this energy changeable in nature. Gemini is an air sign bringing an intellectual and communicative flare to it. Planets that are positioned in this sign are in a state of constant intellectual motion.

Gemini is referred to as "The Twins" and is the sign of the storyteller and communicator. This sign is known for gathering all types of information, being bright and witty with active curiosity. This sign also can be restless, cunning, fickle, gossipy, and two-faced. Gemini is most compatible with Libra, Leo, Aquarius, and Aries. Sagittarius is the opposite sign in the zodiac.

<u>Cancer - June 22 - July 22:</u> Cancer is the fourth sign of the zodiac. It is classified as a cardinal mode and therefore has an initiatory type of energy. It is the first of three water signs in the zodiac; therefore, an emotional or feeling type of nature is associated with it. Planets that are positioned in this sign act in a feeling way, or have a soulful nature about them.

Cancer is also referred to as the "Crab" and is the sign of the protector. Other qualities of this sign are sensitivity, faithfulness, the nurturer, enterprising and shrewdness. The downside qualities to this sign are hypersensitivity, moodiness, devious behavior, and an unforgiving nature. This sign is most compatible with Taurus, Virgo, Scorpio and Pisces. Capricorn is the opposite sign in the zodiac.

<u>Leo - July 23 - August 22:</u> Leo is the fifth sign of the zodiac. It is considered to be a stable or fixed mode, making this energy very grounded or stabilizing in nature. Leo is also a fire sign and has a very spirited or willful type of energy. Planets that are positioned in this sign tend to center and personalize their force.

Leo is also referred to as "The Lion" and is the sign of the ruler. This sign is expansive, caring, and generous in nature. It also has qualities of being flamboyant, intelligent, hardworking and charming. The downside to the Leo energy is being opinionated, overbearing, proud, pompous, and egotistical. Leo is most compatible with Gemini, Aries, Libra, and Sagittarius. Aquarius is the opposite sign in the zodiac from Leo.

<u>Virgo - August 23 - September 22:</u> Virgo is the sixth sign of the zodiac. It is considered to be a flexible or adaptable mode, making this energy changeable in nature. It is also an earth sign giving the energy a rather empirical or experiential way about it. When we combine the qualities of adaptability with an empirical nature, technical efficiency is the outcome. Therefore, planets that are positioned in this sign tend to consider and quantify everything.

Virgo is also referred to as "The Virgin" and is the sign of the critic. There is a sharp intellect, meticulous, and fastidious nature about this sign. However, this sign also has an urge to label, be over-conforming, hypercritical, and overly cautious at times. Virgo is most compatible with

Scorpio, Taurus, Cancer, and Capricorn. The opposite sign in the zodiac is Pisces.

<u>Libra - September 23 - October 22:</u> Libra is the seventh sign of the zodiac. It is considered to be a cardinal mode and exudes an initiatory type of energy. It is also an air sign and therefore has a thinking or intellectual nature about it. Planets that reside in this sign take on a rational and balanced quality.

Libra is also referred to as "The Scales," meaning the scales of justice. The easy-going, diplomatic energy associated with Libra makes this sign an excellent arbitrator when arguments ensue. This sign also can show qualities of indecisiveness, resentfulness, and a frivolous nature. Libra is most compatible with Aquarius, Gemini, Leo, and Sagittarius. Aries is the opposite sign in the zodiac.

<u>Scorpio - October 23 - November 21:</u> Scorpio is the eighth zodiac sign. It is considered to be a stable or fixed energy mode. Scorpio is the second water sign and has an emotional quality about it. When you combine the fixed mode component with the emotional water quality, the outcome is a concealed nature. These are exactly how planets react when positioned in this sign. Scorpio is often tagged with negative energy, as there is a high level of intensity and secretiveness associated with this sign. This is a sign that has a committed, loyal, and determined nature. It also has the energy of deviance, self-pity, hypersensitivity and moodiness. Scorpios are most compatible with Pisces, Cancer, Virgo, and Capricorn. Taurus is its opposite sign in the zodiac.

<u>Sagittarius - November 22 - December 20:</u> Sagittarius is the ninth zodiac sign. It is considered to be an adaptable or flexible sign mode. It is the second fire sign of the zodiac and has a spirited energy associated with it. When you combine the flexible mode with the spirited element, the result is ambition. Planets that reside in this sign take on an ambitious or yearning quality.

Sagittarius is known as "The Archer" and is the sign of the gypsy. This sign is associated with optimism, versatility, open-mindedness, and has visionary qualities. Sagittarius can also have a restless, tactless, and irresponsible nature to it. This sign is most compatible with Aries, Leo, Libra, and Aquarius. Gemini is the opposite sign in the zodiac.

<u>Capricorn - December 21 - January 19:</u> Capricorn is the tenth sign of

the zodiac. It is considered to be a cardinal mode and therefore has an initiatory component to it. It is also the third and final earth sign in the zodiac, making it experiential in nature. Planets that reside in this sign take on a systematic on-going mode of expression.

Capricorn is also known as "The Goat" and is the sign of the achiever. This sign is known for its sense of humor, reliability, determination, and preserving nature. Capricorn can also be rigid, harsh, ruthless, and pessimistic. This sign is most compatible with Taurus, Virgo, Scorpio, and Pisces. The opposite sign in the zodiac is Cancer.

<u>Aquarius - January 20 - February 18:</u> Aquarius is the eleventh sign of the zodiac. It is fixed and stable in its mode and is the third air sign. When the intellectual air quality combines with the fixed mode, the result is a detached energy.

Planets that reside in this sign act in a cool and detached manner. This sign is noted for its independence, quirky, innovative, and humanitarian qualities. Aquarius can also be very unpredictable, eccentric, and rebellious. The most compatible signs are Aries, Gemini, Libra, and Sagittarius. The opposite sign of Aquarius is Leo.

<u>Pisces- February 19- March 20:</u> Pisces is the final sign in the zodiac. It is classified as an adaptable and flexible mode and is the final water sign. The combination of flexibility, with the emotions of a water sign, results in empathy. Planets that reside in this sign take on a feeling and empathic quality. This sign has an artistic, kind, sympathetic, and intuitive nature. It also can have a pessimistic, impractical, unrealistic, fearful, and melancholy type of energy. This sign is most compatible with Taurus, Cancer, Scorpio and Capricorn. The opposite sign in the zodiac is Virgo.

These are the 12 signs of the zodiac in Western Astrology. They are how the prime components (planets) function in a horoscope. In other words, the zodiac signs are how we express our motivations in life.

Eastern Zodiac:

The Chinese animal signs are a twelve-year cycle used for dating the years. It operates under the premise of a cycle, rather than a linear concept that its Western counterpart does. In other words, the dating methods are repeated over time according to a pattern. Like Western Astrology, a chart interpretation is based on many factors besides the "Zodiac Sign." In short, there are four pillars or columns (hour, day, month and year) that are comprised of two sections (Heavenly Stem and Earthly Branch). The Heavenly Stem represents the element (five element theory) and the Earthy Branch represents the archetype animal. From these four pillars various information can be derived about the individual. Below is a list of the archetype animals (zodiac) and their basic descriptions. There are many other facets to the Four Pillars Eastern Astrology method that are not included in this book.

Rat- 1912, 1924, 1936, 1948, 1960, 1972, 1984, 1996, 2008, 2020: Individuals born under this animal sign tend to be creative, charming, generous, and work hard to achieve their goals. They are very ambitious and tend to be successful in life. Rats can also be lustful, pessimistic, quick-tempered, and overly critical. They are most compatible with people born in the years of the Dragon, Monkey, and Ox.

Ox- 1913, 1925, 1937, 1949, 1961, 1973, 1985, 1997, 2009, 2021: Those born in the year of the Ox tend to be patient, preserving, methodical, hard-working, are mentally and physically alert, and can inspire confidence in others. The Ox can also be stubborn, obstinate and hate to fail at anything in life. They are most compatible with people born in the year of the Snake, Rooster, and Rat.

Tiger- 1914, 1926, 1938, 1950, 1962, 1974, 1986, 1998, 2010, 2022: Those who are born in the year of the Tiger are wise, compassionate, sensitive, courageous, and powerful. They also have a tendency to be short-tempered, proud, difficulty with decision-making, and aggressive behavior. They are most compatible with those born in the year of the Horse, Dragon, and Dog.

Appendix

Rabbit- 1915, 1927, 1939, 1951, 1963, 1975, 1987, 1999, 2011, 2023:
Those born under this animal sign are gentle in nature, friendly, intelligent, articulate, talented, very calm, and virtuous. The Rabbit can also be rather fickle and secretive. This animal sign is most compatible with those born in the year of the Sheep, Dog, and Pig.

Dragon- 1916, 1928, 1940, 1952, 1964, 1976, 1988, 2000, 2012, 2024:
The Dragon energy is proud, powerful, healthy, energetic, confident, courageous, and honest. The Dragon can be aggressive, uncompromising, self-centered, and short-tempered. The animal signs most compatible with the Dragon are the Rat, Snake, Monkey, and Rooster.

Snake- 1917, 1929, 1941, 1953, 1965, 1977, 1989, 2001, 2013, 2025:
The Snake energy is one of great wisdom, determination, intensity, and passion. Snakes are financially secure and show sensitivity to others. The Snake can be stingy, vain, secretive, and selfish. They are most compatible with the Ox and Rooster.

Horse- 1918, 1930, 1942, 1954, 1966, 1978, 1990, 2002, 2014, 2026:
The Horse is elegant, sociable, keen high-spirited, popular, independent, and skillful with money. The downside to the Horse personality is they can be obstinate, anger easily, and rarely listen to advice. The Horse is most compatible with those born in the year of the Tiger, Dog, and Sheep.

Sheep- 1919, 1931, 1943, 1955, 1967, 1979, 1991, 2003, 2015, 2027:
The Sheep has a graceful, obedient, and spiritual nature about them. Sheep are very creative in the arts and passionate in what they do. The Sheep personality can be shy, timid, and pessimistic. They are most compatible with those born in the year of the Rabbit, Pig, and Horse.

Monkey- 1920, 1932, 1944, 1956, 1968, 1980, 1992, 2004, 2016, 2028:
The Monkey is ingenious, curious, and resourceful. They can be very inventive and have a great desire to obtain knowledge. The Monkey can also be very strong-willed, easily distracted, and impulsive with their actions. The Monkey is most compatible with the Dragon and Rat.

Rooster- 1921, 1933, 1945, 1957, 1969, 1981, 1993, 2005, 2017, 2029:
The Rooster is a visionary, versatile in nature, and a deep thinker. They prefer to be busy, and because of this, tend to overextend themselves. The energy of the Rooster is one of eccentricity and adventure. They can be selfish, ostentatious, and have a tendency to be a loner. The Rooster is most compatible with the Ox, Snake, and Dragon.

Dog- 1922, 1934, 1946, 1958, 1970, 1982, 1994, 2006, 2018, 2030:
The Dog is about loyalty, honesty, respect and inspiration. They have a great ability to stay focused and are straightforward in their actions. Dogs can also be selfish, demanding, stubborn, and rather terse at times. They are most compatible with those born in the year of the Horse, Tiger, and Rabbit.

Pig- 1923, 1935, 1947, 1959, 1971, 1983, 1995, 2007, 2019, 2031:
The Pig has a serious but genuine disposition. The Pig has great fortitude, is honest, conscientious, loyal, and extremely knowledgeable. The downside of the Pig is their quick-temper, impatient, and inflexible nature. They are most compatible with Rabbits and Sheep.

These are the twelve archetype animals of the Eastern Zodiac. Some of these animals are more compatible in nature than others as mentioned in the animal descriptions. These high levels of compatibility are based on the position of the animals around the zodiac. When they form a trine, it is the most balanced and stable configuration. These configurations are seen with the following animals.

First Trine	Second Trine	Third Trine
o Rat (North)	o Ox (Northeast)	o Rabbit (East)
o Dragon (East by Southeast)	o Snake (Southeast)	o Sheep (South by Southwest)
o Monkey (Southwest)	o Rooster (West)	o Pig (North by Northwest)
*These animals are very supportive to one another in understanding their individual ambitions.	* These are considered to be the most intellectual and determined animals of the Chinese zodiac.	* These animals are the most sympathetic and compassionate of the zodiac.

Appendix

There are other levels of compatibility between the animals with the most challenging being those that are in direct opposition to each other on the Chinese compass. Even though this position between the animals constitutes a clash and can be the result of life's greatest challenges, it is usually what creates our greatest accomplishments. The most incompatible animal configurations are as follows.

<u>Clash</u>
Rat (North) and Horse (South)

<u>Clash</u>
Ox (North by Northeast)
Sheep (South by Southwest)

<u>Clash</u>
Tiger (Northeast)
Monkey (Southwest)

<u>Clash</u>
Rabbit (East)
Rooster (West)

<u>Clash</u>
Dragon (East by Southeast)
Dog (West by Northwest)

<u>Clash</u>
Snake (Southeast)
Pig (Northwest)

Analyzing the four pillars chart takes years of study and practice. Studying the interactions between the Earthly Branches and their associated elements with the Heavenly Stems and their designated elements along with the hidden elements in the chart is the basis for the interpretive process. A hierarchy of defining elements within the chart also aids in the discovery process.

About The Author

Mary Jane Kasliner

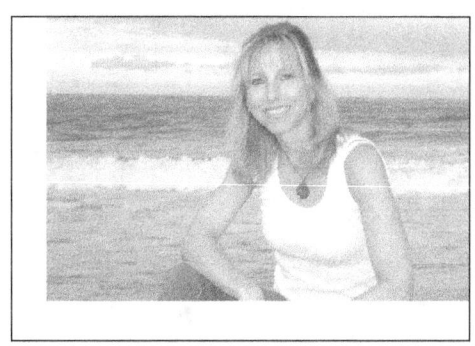

Mary Jane (MJ) Kasliner, is an author, teacher, lifestyle master, and creator of Codes of Creation in Movement®.

Since 1985, MJ has dedicated her career to helping others improve their health and well-being. She started her professional life as a Respiratory Therapist and Dental Hygienist before she made the radical shift into the world of Metaphysics.

Her big career move occurred in 2002, and she has been astounded ever since by the transformation of her readers and clients who incorporate her lifestyle strategies into their lives.

Mary Jane graduated from Skidmore College with a degree in Health Science and from Union College with a degree in Applied Sciences. She studied Western Feng Shui at the De Amicis School in Philadelphia and Classical Feng Shui at the New York School of Feng Shui and Feng Shui Institute of London. In 2008, Mary Jane completed her 200-hour national teacher training program in Hatha Yoga at the Center of Health and Healing and Personal Revolution Barron Baptiste Program at Yoga Bliss. Several years afterward, she completed her Mastery of Meditation Program with Master Anmol Mehta. Mary Jane also completed Chakra Therapy certification from Bodhi Yoga Center in Utah and additional training in New York, New Jersey, and India.

Mary Jane believes in giving back to the world for human welfare. MJ was honored to be a part of Sean Corn's Off the Mat and Into the World humanitarian effort to Uganda where she raised thousands of dollars for orphaned children due to war and AIDS.

Mary Jane has received worldwide media coverage from the Associated Press for her work. She has been interviewed on TV and radio, author of nine books, two online training programs, a DIY Power of Attraction publication, and a lifestyle coach in her Codes of Creation Mastermind System.

Mary Jane loves to play golf and travel in her spare time. She can be contacted at www.mjkasliner.com

About The Illustrator

Ann Curch Gagliano

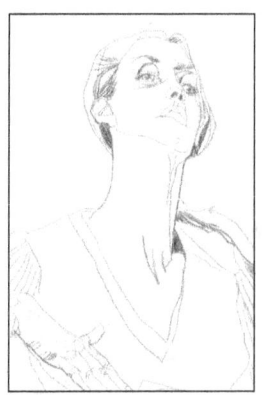

Ann Curch Gagliano is both an Artist and Mother. She graduated from Parsons School of Design in New York City where she earned a Bachelors in Fine Arts in Illustrative Design. In her early career she worked in advertising creating storyboards, product designs, and print ads for some of the world's largest companies. Her fine art work has been exhibited throughout the state of New Jersey and New York where she has won several awards on a local and national level. Ann's subject matter to date is primarily figurative drawings and paintings of the human form. Her clientele includes corporate, small business, residential, and freelance work. She lives in New Jersey with her husband, two children and their dog "TTmom."

Resources & Bibliography

Consulting Services

Mary Jane Kasliner is a Yoga - Feng Shui Lifestyle Master that utilizes the age-old principles of Feng Shui and Yoga. What we experience in life is reflected energetically by our thoughts and surroundings. When we change our thoughts and what's happening around us in a positive way, we reshape what happens in our lives.

Her approach is simple: by empowering your surroundings, you empower yourself. Your desires are sown and you are able to express your unique gifts to the world. Yoga is the finishing touch that can foster your journey to creating a life well-lived from a higher state of being. Mary Jane invites you to explore her website (www.mjkasliner.com) and review all of her offerings.

Electro-Magnetic Devices

Today, in this fast paced technology oriented 21st century, we have removed ourselves from nature. As a result, we have become less aware of the energies that can impact our bodies. These energies are referred to as "Electro-stress" and are created by man-made structures such as high-tension wires, cell towers, televisions, computers, cell phones, microwaves, and other household appliances. The products below are distributed from Biomagnetic Research Company. They are made from a unique composition of space-age ceramics that can absorb harmful electromagnetic radiations and rebroadcast them out into a cleaner form.

- Crystal Catalyst Bead®
- Cellular Phone Tab
- Electronic Smog Buster
- Twelve Point Resonator
- Tri-pak Resonator
- Crystal Catalyst Pendants

Natural Air Purifiers

Salt lamps and salt candles are a natural way to purify air in the home. The sodium and chloride (two elements of salt) create a bond, that when heated, causes the sodium and chloride ions to break apart. In the process, the chloride ion takes an extra electron from the outer shell of the sodium atom making it negatively charged. Pollutants in the air from bacteria, viruses, allergens, and electromagnetic discharges are all positively charged. Because positive and negative charges are attracted to each other, the bad positive ions surround the good negative ions and attach to it. As a result, the particle becomes heavy and falls to the ground where it then can be vacuumed away. For further information on salt purifiers use the World Wide Web.

Bibliography

Art Explosion. Royalty Free Clip Art: (Nova Development Corporation, 2004).

Chia, Mantak, Dirk Oellibrandt. *Taoist Astral Healing*. Destiny Books, Vermont, 2004.

Chin, K., Peter. *15 Ways To Find A Happier You*. Rainbow Tai-Chi Productions, 1996.

Collins, Kathryn,Terah. *The Western Guide to Feng Shui*. Hay House, Inc., California, 1996.

Cowan, David. *Safe As Houses*. Gateway Books. 2002.

DeAmicis, Drs. Ralph & Lahni. *Feng Shui and the Tango*. Cuore Libre Multimedia Publishing, PA, 2004.

Dyer, Wayne. *Manifest Your Destiny*. Harper Collins Publishers, Inc., New York, 1997.

Fahrnow, Maria, Sator, Gunther. *Feng Shui And The 5-Element Kitchen*. Silverback Books, Inc. 2000.

Gerber, Dr. Richard. *Vibrational Medicine*. Bear & Company. Rochester, VT, 1996.

Green, Roger. *The I Ching Workbook*. New Holland Publishers (Australia) Pty Ltd., 2004.

Hall, Judy. *The Illustrated Guide To Crystals*. Sterling Publishing Co., Inc., New York, 2000.

Hartdegen, Stephen, O.F.M., S.S.L. *Holy Bible*. World Publishing Inc. 1987.

Hudson, John. *Instant Meditation For Stress Relief*. Anness Publishing Limited, London, 1996.

Hwa, Tsung, Jou. *The Tao of Tai-Chi*. Tai-Chi Foundation, 1980.

Jones, Larissa. *Aromatherapy: for Body, Mind, and Spirit.* Evergreen Aromatherapy, Utah, 2001.

Kasliner, Mary Jane, BS. co-author, *Love, Happiness And Feng Shui.* Booksurge Publishing, LLC., South Carolina, 2004.

Katzman, Shoshanna. *Qigong For Staying Young.* Avery Books, New York, 2003.

Kingston, Karen. *Creating Sacred Space With Feng Shui.* Broadway Books, New York, 1997.

Kwok, Man-Ho, Joanne O'Brien. *The Elements of Feng Shui.* Barnes & Noble Inc., New York, 1997.

Lakhovsky, George. *The Secret Life.* London, 1939.

Lawlor, Robert. *Sacred Geometry.* Thames and Hudson Ltd., London, 1982.

LeCouteur, Don. *Client Centered Astrology.* Copyright Don LeCouteur, 2001.

Legge, James. *The Great Plan.* Clarindon Press, Oxford 1893.

Lim, Jes, Dr. *Feng Shui & Your Health.* Times Books International, Singapore, 1999.

Linn, Denise. *Feng Shui For The Soul.* Hay House, Inc. Calsbad, California, 1999.

Richards, Rick. *The Human Chakra System.* World-Wide Web, 2006.

SantoPietro, Nancy. *Feng Shui and Health.* Three Rivers Press, New York, 2002.

Sachs, Robert. *Nine Star Ki.* Vega, London, 2001.

Soltes, Fiona. *Oils Of The Ancients.* Asbury Park Press Newspaper, New Jersey, March, 2004.

Shen, Zaihong. Feng Shui: *Harmonizing Your Inner & Outer Space.* Dorling Kindersley Publishing, Inc. N.Y., 2001.

Tanzer, Elliot. *Choose The Best House For You.* Elliot Jay Tanzer, California, 2003.

Toy, Fiona. *Auras and Chakras: Harnessing The Energy Within.* Barnes & Noble Books, New York, 2002.

Walters, Derek. *Chinese Astrology.* Watkins Publishing, London, 2002.

Wong, Eva. *Feng Shui: The Ancient Wisdom of Harmonious Living for Modern Times.* Shambhala Publications, Inc. Boston, 1996.

Yang, Wang, Dr., Jon Sandifer. *The Authentic I Ching.* Watkins Publishing, London 2003.

* Key resources for the compilation of this work were based on Mary Jane Kasliner's feng shui educational notes. Schools attended include: The DeAmicis School of Western Feng Shui, New York School of Feng Shui, Feng Shui Institute in London, and the CCA School of Western Astrology in Oregon.

Additional Notes

<u>Chapter Beginning Quotes</u>: All quotes provided in chapter fronts, beginning, and end of book are granted permission by the "Fair Use" act.

<u>Chapter 3</u>: Page 44- 46 "Personality Descriptions of Trigrams" quoted resource – 9 Star Ki by Robert Sachs. Author contacted and permission granted.

<u>Chapter 4</u>: Major source referenced - Safe As Houses by David Cowan. Author contacted and permission granted.

<u>Chapter 5</u>: Problematic designs with cures - resource referenced with quoted notes – Choose The Best House For You by Elliot Tanzer. Author contacted and permission granted. * Many other Feng Shui resources contain similar information including Feng Shui training programs author attended.

<u>Chapter 6</u>: References made from the book: Manifest Your Destiny by Wayne Dyer – permission granted by Hay House Inc.

<u>Chapter 8</u>: Page 169 quoted resource – Feng Shui For The Soul by Denise Linn. Author contacted and permission granted.

* The aforementioned were key resources in portions of this book. I express my deepest gratitude to these authors and others referenced in my bibliography for their commitment to the Feng Shui profession and helping others to live at a higher energy level. I highly recommend their books along with the listed bibliography of books.

"A home is not dead but living, and like all living things must obey the laws of nature by constantly changing."

Carl Larsson

www.ingramcontent.com/pod-product-compliance
Lightning Source LLC
Chambersburg PA
CBHW071354290426
44108CB00014B/1540